SLEEP – PHYSIOLOGY, FUNCTIONS, DREAMING AND DISORDERS SERIES

NARCOLEPSY: SYMPTOMS, CAUSES AND DIAGNOSIS

SLEEP – PHYSIOLOGY, FUNCTIONS, DREAMING AND DISORDERS SERIES

Narcolepsy: Symptoms, Causes and Diagnosis
Guillermo Santos and Lautar Villalba (Editors)
2010. ISBN: 978-1-60876-645-1

SLEEP – PHYSIOLOGY, FUNCTIONS, DREAMING AND DISORDERS SERIES

NARCOLEPSY: SYMPTOMS, CAUSES AND DIAGNOSIS

GUILLERMO SANTOS
AND
LAUTAR VILLALBA
EDITORS

Nova Science Publishers, Inc.
New York

For permission to use material from this book please contact us:
Telephone 631-231-7269; Fax 631-231-8175
Web Site: http://www.novapublishers.com

Library of Congress Cataloging-in-Publication Data

Narcolepsy : symptoms, causes, and diagnosis / editors, Guillermo Santos and Lautar Villalba.
p. ; cm.
Includes bibliographical references and index.
ISBN 978-1-60876-645-1 (hardcover : alk. paper)
1. Narcolepsy. I. Santos, Guillermo. II. Villalba, Lautar.
[DNLM: 1. Narcolepsy. WM 188 N2225 2009]
RC549.N373 2009
616.8'498--dc22

2009044331

Published by Nova Science Publishers, Inc. † New York

Contents

Preface

Narcolepsy is a clinical syndrome defined by four symptoms: a compliant excessive sleepiness, a sudden bilateral loss of postural muscle tone, sleep paralysis and hypnagogic hallucinations. When cataplexy is predominant, narcolepsy can be misdiagnosed as syncope or drop attacks. The authors of this book discuss how to correctly diagnosis narcolepsy and how to avoid certain pitfalls which would lead to erroneous treatments due to the misdiagnosis. Moreover, this book examines the role exerted by obesity in the pathophysiological mechanisms of narcolepsy. This book underlines the importance of body weight as a factor influencing the narcolepsy, indicating also the possible therapeutic strategies by modifications of eating behavior. In addition, modafinil is a mild, wake-promoting stimulant that is pharmacologically distinct from other central nervous system stimulants. This book provides an overview of modafinil's effects on human and animal behavior and in the brain. Other chapters assess narcolepsy in children, the influences of orexin A in the pathophysiological mechanisms of narcolepsy and the prevalence of periodic leg movements (PLM) in people who suffer from narcolepsy.

Chapter I - Human narcolepsy is thought to be caused by the degeneration of orexin (hypocretin)-containing neurons. There are two genetically engineered mice models of orexin deficiency to study possible roles of intrinsic orexin in physiological functions. One is the prepro-orexin knockout mouse that was developed by a conventional knockout technique and another is the orexin neuron-ablated mouse. The latter was developed using a transgenic technique by introducing a truncated Machado-Joseph disease gene product (ataxin-3) with an expanded polyglutamine stretch under the control of the orexin-promoter. Although the cause of orexin deficiency in both mice models is not the same to the human's (presumably autoimmune), both mice expressed narcoleptic phenotype showing importance of orexin in sleep/wake regulation.

The authors studied autonomic functions in these mutant animals and found abnormalities in vigilance state- and emotional state-dependent adjustment of the central autonomic regulation on circulation and respiration. These are summarized as follows. 1) Orexin-deficient mice show an attenuated hypercapnic ventilatory response during the awake but not during the sleep period, whereas basal ventilation remained normal, irrespective of the vigilance state. Orexin supplementation remedied the defect, and the administration of an orexin receptor antagonist to wild-type mice mimicked the abnormality. 2) Orexin-deficient mice also showed frequent sleep apneas and loss of repetitive intermittent hypoxia-induced ventilatory long-term facilitation. 3) Orexin-deficient mice exposed to a stressor presented an attenuated fight-or-flight response, including increases in respiration and blood pressure and stress-induced analgesia. 4) Both hypercapnic and emotional stimulation activates orexinergic neurons in the wild-type mice. Hence, it is likely that the orexin system is one of the essential modulators required for orchestrating the neural circuits controlling autonomic functions and behaviors.

Chapter II - Modafinil is a mild, wake-promoting stimulant that is pharmacologically distinct from other central nervous system stimulants. Modafinil is approved in the United States for the treatment of narcolepsy and has been demonstrated to be effective and well-tolerated. Modafinil also has been approved for use in treating shift work sleep disorder and as an adjunctive treatment for obstructive sleep apnea/hypopnea syndrome. Similar to other stimulants, modafinil increases arousal and has cognitive benefits. Beyond managing sleep disorders, modafinil has been used to manage the symptoms of Attention-Deficit Hyperactivity Disorder, depression, schizophrenia, and addiction to cocaine and amphetamines. The findings with human subjects have been supported by basic animal behavioral research. Despite modafinil's numerous clinical uses, its mechanism of action in the brain is unclear: Modafinil interacts with multiple targets in the central nervous system—dopamine, norepinephrine, serotonin and orexin receptors—associated with modafinil's clinical and behavioral effects. This chapter offers an overview of modafinil's effects on human and animal behavior and in the brain.

Chapter III - Narcolepsy is a clinical syndrome defined by four symptoms: a compliant excessive sleepiness; a sudden bilateral loss of postural muscle tone or a sudden muscle weakness, often subsequent to an intense emotion (Cataplexy); sleep paralysis; hypnagogic hallucinations. The syndrome can be idiopathic or secondary to other medical condition (neurological diseases, other sleep disorders or drugs abuse). In the presence of pathognomonic clinical criteria, diagnosis is confirmed by video-polysomnography (vPSG), Multiple Sleep latency Test (MLST). The presence of HLA-DR2 and low hypocretin values in cerebrospinal fluid can support this diagnosis.

According to the International Classification of Sleep Disorders (ICSD-2v) the authors can distinguish Narcolepsy into two major groups: Narcolepsy with or without cataplexy.

The main difference between the two entities is the absence of typical cataplexy and the necessity in narcolepsy without cataplexy to confirm the clinical diagnosis by nocturnal vPSG followed by MSLT showing two or more sleep onset REM periods.

Narcolepsy with Cataplexy is often misdiagnosed as a psychiatric condition or as an epilepsy variant or other form of hypersomnia (i.e. sleep apnea syndrome, hypersomnia due to depression). When cataplexy is predominant, Narcolepsy can be misdiagnosed as syncope, drop attacks, atonic attacks or attacks of a histrionic nature. Instead when sleep paralysis and/or hypnagogic hallucinations are predominant symptoms, narcolepsy can be confounded for psychological/psychiatric disease, but also for other REM parasomnia.

Narcolepsy without cataplexy may overlap with idiopathic hypersomnia.

In conclusion a correct diagnosis of narcolepsy is important since this syndrome has a good outcome and, usually, improves with specific drugs (modafinil, sodium oxybate, SSRI, tricyclic antidepressants). Moreover, erroneous treatments due to a misdiagnosis can precipitate or exacerbate the symptoms of Narcolepsy.

Chapter IV - Childhood narcolepsy can be a key to our understanding of the pathogenesis of this disease. The most recent research has been focused on the possibility of autoimmune-mediated destruction of hypocretin/orexin-containing neurons particularly in children and adolescents, and on early diagnosis. However, the diagnosis of childhood narcolepsy is more difficult than in later life, particularly for the specific symptoms appearing in early childhood. Daytime sleepiness has a longer duration in toddlers and preschool children and cataplectic attacks are often mistaken for astatic-myoclonic epileptic seizures. Young patients seem less disturbed by cataplexy than adults; lacking self-awareness, they continue to watch cartoons, conduct other activities or joke even in the presence of multiple repetitive attacks. A semipermanent state of facial muscle weakness with occasional exacerbations is a marked feature there. Toddlers and preschool children are unable to express states of hypnagogic/hypnopompic hallucinations and/or sleep paralysis in their own words, hence, clinical evaluation of narcolepsy is particularly critical as normative data for MSLT corresponding to different children's age are not available. Attention should, therefore, be paid to sleep diary, pediatric sleepiness scale, actigraphy, long-term polysomnographic monitoring, human leukocyte tests and hypocretin evaluation. Complementary methods including neuroimaging and genetic tests are necessary to exclude secondary (symptomatic) cases, particularly if cataplectic attacks predominate. The treatment and management of pediatric cases require a specific approach. These reasons contributed to the development of the international PHEA (Physical Health Executive Agency) project devoted to rare pediatric neurological diseases (nEUroped) covering also childhood narcolepsy. Ten European countries participate in this research centered mainly on patient-related optimization of medical care (diagnosis and therapy), on interaction and collaboration between centers, patients and their family members, and on recommendations for young narcoleptics′ psychological and social needs.

Chapter V - Many patients with narcolepsy complain about cognitive problems, in addition to the characteristic symptoms of increased tiredness and sleepiness. Neuropsychological researches have mainly focused on memory and attentional abilities. In contrast to self-reports, standardized assessment of memory abilities yielded intact or mild deficit of short- and long- term memory. Conversely, attentional deficits are frequently reported mostly if attention has to be maintained over longer periods of time and if the tasks require a higher degree of cognitive control.

Chapter VI - Orexin A is produced almost exclusively in the dorsal and lateral hypothalamus but its projection is widespread within the brain and plays important roles. This system plays a crucial role in the regulation of sleep and wakefulness. On the other hand, orexin A exerts a strong influence on thermoregulation and eating behavior. This peptide could control sleep/wakefulness states throughout modifications of body temperature and eating behavior. The influences of orexin A in the pathophysiological mechanisms of narcolepsy are discussed.

Chapter VII - The causes of sleep disruption in patients with narcolepsy are not clearly identified. Possible causes include daytime sleep through planned or unplanned naps, impairment of the delta-wave generating mechanisms, and comorbid sleep disorders such as sleep disordered breathing and periodic leg movements (PLMs). PLMs have been proposed as one of the causes of increased arousal in narcolepsy. Two recent controlled studies have demonstrated increased prevalence of PLMs in narcoleptics compared to controls with an impact on sleep latency on multiple sleep latency test. At the present, the contribution of PLMs to the perceived sleep quality and daytime sleepiness in narcolepsy patients is not clear. The observation that PLMs arousals were significantly higher in the PLMs group suggests that reducing the frequency of PLMs may improve sleep architecture. The pathophysiology of narcolepsy may involve an abnormal cholinergic-dopaminergic interaction. Pharmacological agents that decrease dopaminergic release, such as gamma-hydroxybutyrate and neuroleptic-D2 receptor antagonists, have been shown to worsen PLMs. Additionally, dysfunction in the hypocretin/dopaminergic system is likely to be one of the mechanisms involved in the pathophysiology of narcolepsy, with alterations in arousal systems but also in sleep-related motor activation with a large amount of PLMS.

Chapter VIII - This expert commentary reports the role exerted by obesity in the pathophysiological mechanisms of narcolepsy. Generally, the narcolepsy is described almost exclusively a neurological disease, while the role of nutritional and metabolic factors is almost neglected. The influences of body weight control and obesity are not sufficiently underlined. A search on "PubMed" (April 2009) with the words "narcolepsy and obesity" reports only 137 articles, while the search of the words "narcolepsy and body weight" produces 93 papers. This commentary underlines the importance of body weight as factor influencing the narcolepsy, indicating also the possible therapeutic strategies by modifications of eating behavior.

In: Nacrolepsy: Symptoms, Causes...
Editors: G. Santos et al. pp. 1-33
ISBN: 978-1-60876-645-1

Chapter I

Autonomic Malfunctions in Mice Model of Narcolepsy

***Tomoyuki Kuwaki*[1*] *and Wei Zhang*[2]**
[1]Department of Physiology, Kagoshima University Graduate School of Medical & Dental Sciences, Kagoshima 890-8544, Japan.
[2]Department of Neurology, University of Iowa, IA 52242-1009, USA.

Abstract

Human narcolepsy is thought to be caused by the degeneration of orexin (hypocretin)-containing neurons. There are two genetically engineered mice models of orexin deficiency to study possible roles of intrinsic orexin in physiological functions. One is the prepro-orexin knockout mouse that was developed by a conventional knockout technique and another is the orexin neuron-ablated mouse. The latter was developed using a transgenic technique by introducing a truncated Machado-Joseph disease gene product (ataxin-3) with an expanded polyglutamine stretch under the control of the orexin-promoter. Although the cause of orexin deficiency in both mice models is not the same to the human's (presumably autoimmune), both mice expressed

* Corresponding author: Department of Physiology, Kagoshima University Graduate School of Medical & Dental Sciences, Sakuragaoka 8-35-1, Kagoshima 890-8544, Japan, E-mail: kuwaki@m3.kufm.kagoshima-u.ac.jp, Phone: +81-99-275-5227, Fax: +81-99-275-5231,

narcoleptic phenotype showing importance of orexin in sleep/wake regulation.

We studied autonomic functions in these mutant animals and found abnormalities in vigilance state- and emotional state-dependent adjustment of the central autonomic regulation on circulation and respiration. These are summarized as follows. 1) Orexin-deficient mice show an attenuated hypercapnic ventilatory response during the awake but not during the sleep period, whereas basal ventilation remained normal, irrespective of the vigilance state. Orexin supplementation remedied the defect, and the administration of an orexin receptor antagonist to wild-type mice mimicked the abnormality. 2) Orexin-deficient mice also showed frequent sleep apneas and loss of repetitive intermittent hypoxia-induced ventilatory long-term facilitation. 3) Orexin-deficient mice exposed to a stressor presented an attenuated fight-or-flight response, including increases in respiration and blood pressure and stress-induced analgesia. 4) Both hypercapnic and emotional stimulation activates orexinergic neurons in the wild-type mice. Hence, it is likely that the orexin system is one of the essential modulators required for orchestrating the neural circuits controlling autonomic functions and behaviors.

1. Introduction

1.1. Autonomic Malfunction in Human Narcolepsy

There are only a few reports describing autonomic regulation in narcolepsy patients. Sachs and Kaijser (1982) reported that never medicated narcoleptic patients showed attenuated autonomic reflexes (changes in blood pressure and heart rate) in handgrip test and Valsalva's maneuver, but not in face immersion test or orthostatic standing. Because some but not all reflexes had been disturbed, they proposed intact peripheral nerves and a localization of the defect to the central nervous system. Basal blood pressure in narcolepsy patients is rather controversial. The same author reported normal blood pressure and heart rate at rest before the autonomic testing (Sachs et al., 1982). However, Guilleminault (1993) reported that withdrawal of medication with amphetamine for four weeks significantly decreased blood pressure in narcoleptic patients, indicating low blood pressure otherwise taking a central stimulant. Both of sympathetic and parasympathetic basal activities seemed to be decreased since heart rate and blood pressure variabilities were significantly decreased in untreated narcoleptic patients (Fronczek et al., 2008). As to regulation of breathing, narcolepsy patients had frequent sleep apneas compared with healthy controls (Chokroverty, 1986) or with idiopathic CNS hypersomnia (Baker et al., 1986). We feel that systematic re-investigation about autonomic regulation in narcoleptic patients is needed, since most of these reports cited here appeared before 2000 when deficiency of orexin had been revealed as the cause of narcolepsy (Thannickal et al., 2000).

1.2. Animal Model of Narcolepsy

There are two genetically engineered mice models of orexin deficiency to study possible roles of intrinsic orexin in physiological functions. One is the prepro-orexin knockout (ORX-KO) mouse that was developed by a conventional knockout technique (Chemelli et al., 1999) and another is the orexin neuron-ablated mouse (Hara et al., 2001). The latter was developed using a transgenic technique by introducing a truncated Machado-Joseph disease gene product (ataxin-3) with an expanded polyglutamine stretch under the control of the orexin-promoter. In these orexin/ataxin-3 transgenic (ORX/ATX-Tg) mice, orexinergic neurons are selectively and postnataly degenerated, and reach >99% loss at the age of 4 months (Hara et al., 2001). Orexinergic neurons contain not only orexin but also other neuropeptides or modulatory factors such as dynorphin (Chou et al., 2001), galanin (Hakansson et al., 1999), glutamate (Abrahamson et al., 2001; Rosin et al., 2003), and nitric oxide (Cheng et al., 2003). These substances also disappear in ORX/ATX-Tg mice.

Although the cause of orexin deficiency in both mice models is not the same to the human's (presumably autoimmune), both mice expressed narcoleptic phenotype showing importance of orexin in sleep/wake regulation.

1.3. Orexin (Hypocretin)

Orexins (orexin-A and orexin-B), also known as hypocretins (hypocretin 1 and hypocretin 2, respectively), are hypothalamic neuropeptides (de Lecea et al., 1998; Sakurai et al., 1998). They are cleaved from a common precursor molecule, prepro-orexin (130 residues), forming orexin-A (33 amino acids) and orexin-B (28 amino acids) (Sakurai et al., 1998; Willie et al., 2001). The orexin-1 receptor has a 10-fold selectivity for orexin-A whereas the orexin-2 receptor, which was identified by database search with amino acid sequence of the orexin-1 receptor, binds to orexin-A and -B with equal affinity (Sakurai et al., 1998; Willie et al., 2001).

Although orexins were first described as hypothalamic neuropeptides facilitating appetite (Sakurai et al., 1998) and consciousness (Chemelli et al., 1999), later studies showed that orexins also modulate motivation (Harris et al., 2006), analgesia (Yamamoto et al., 2002; Watanabe et al., 2005), and autonomic regulation of the cardiovascular (Shirasaka et al., 1999; Dun et al., 2000; Zhang et al., 2006b), respiratory (Young et al., 2005; Zhang et al., 2005), and neuroendocrine (Jászberényi et al., 2000) systems.

1.4. Anatomical Evidence Supporting Orexinergic Modulation of Autonomic Homeostasis

The location of orexin containing cell bodies is restricted to the lateral hypothalamic area (LHA), perifornical area (PFA), and dorsomedial hypothalamus (DMH). Conversely, orexin-containing nerve terminals and receptors are widely distributed in the hypothalamus, thalamus, cerebral cortex, circumventricular organs, brain stem, cerebellum, and spinal cord, suggesting that orexinergic neurons have widespread connections with other regions in the brain (Elias et al., 1998; Nambu et al., 1999). Specifically, cardiorespiratory-related sites that receive orexinergic innervation are the nucleus tractus solitarius; Pre-Bötzinger complex; periaqueductal gray; rostral ventrolateral medulla; intermediolateral cell column of the spinal cord; retrotrapezoid, hypoglossal, raphe, and phrenic nuclei (Figure 1) (Peyron et al., 1998; Dun et al., 2000; Antunes et al., 2001; Fung et al., 2001; Smith et al., 2002; Volgin et al., 2002; Geerling et al., 2003; Berthoud et al., 2005; Dergacheva et al., 2005; Young et al., 2005; Rosin et al., 2006). Approximately 50% of hypothalamic neurons that innervate both the sympathetic efferent and motor cortex or medial prefrontal cortex which is implicated in mental stress showed orexin-like immunoreactivity (Krout et al., 2003; Krout et al., 2005).

Moreover, orexinergic neurons receive inputs from the regulatory sites of sleep/awake and emotional stress such as ventrolateral preoptic area; locus coeruleus; dorsal raphe; amygdala; bed nucleus of stria terminalis (BNST); suprachiasmatic and tuberomammillary nuclei (Sakurai et al., 2005b; Yoshida et al., 2006; Zhang et al., 2009). Numerous neurons in the amygdala, a putative center for biological value judgment (Pitkanen et al., 1997), are retrogradely labeled by cholera toxin B subunit injected into the PFA (Yoshida et al., 2006) and by the trans-synaptic transport of tetanus toxin expressed by the orexin promoter (Sakurai et al., 2005b).

These anatomic feature establishes the basis for a contribution by orexin to a link between the regulatory systems of consciousness (sleep/awake or emotional stress) and of unconscious homeostatic reflexes (Figure 1).

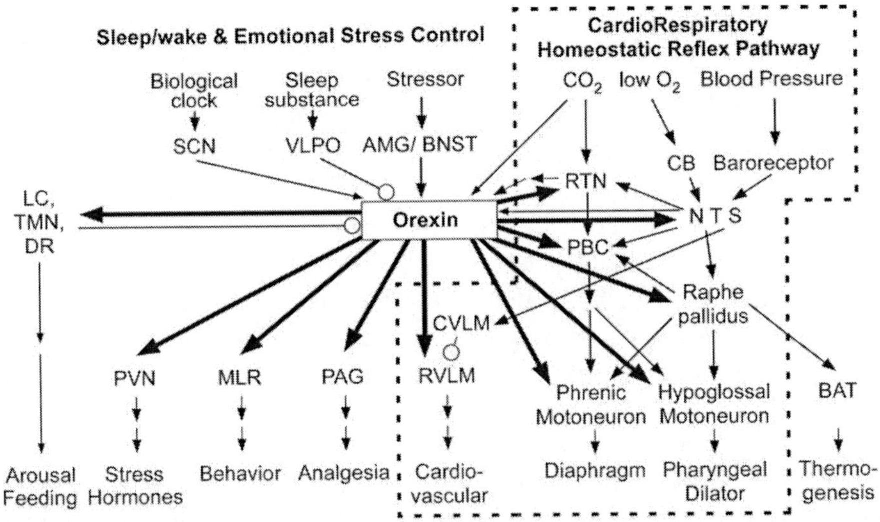

Figure 1. Proposed pathways for the modification of autonomic homeostasis by orexin. Many nuclei in the homeostatic reflex pathway against the changes in CO_2, O_2, and blood pressure receive projections from orexinergic neurons in the hypothalamus (thick line). Simultaneously, orexinergic connections are engaged in sleep/wake regulation and emotional stress-induced autonomic and behavioral changes. Arrows indicate a probable excitatory connection and circles indicate an inhibitory connection. Neurons without direct connection to/from orexinergic neurons are omitted for simplicity. Abbreviations: AMG, amygdala; BAT, brown adipose tissue; BNST, bed nucleus of stria terminalis; CB, carotid body; CVLM, caudal ventrolateral medulla; DR, dorsal raphe; LC, locus coeruleus; MLR, medullary locomotor region; NTS, nucleus tractus solitarius; PAG, periaqueductal gray; PBC, Pre-Bötzinger complex; PVN, paraventricular nucleus; RTN, retrotrapezoid nucleus; RVLM, rostral ventrolateral medulla; SCN, suprachiasmatic nucleus; TMN, tuberomammillary nucleus; VLPO, ventrolateral preoptic nucleus.

2. Autonomic Malfunctions in Orexin Deficient Mice

2.1. Breathing Regulation across Vigilance States

Basal respiration and respiratory reflex regulations are considerably different during the awake and sleep states (Douglas, 2000; Krieger, 2000). For example, tidal volume is largest during awake periods, decreases by 20–30% during slow-wave sleep (SWS), and decreases further during rapid-eye-movement (REM) sleep. Respiratory frequency decreases during SWS and is lower than that during quiet wakefulness (QW); however, respiratory frequency does not decrease during REM sleep. Consequently, the rank order of minute ventilation is QW > SWS ≥ REM. In addition, both the rhythm and amplitude of ventilation are extremely regular during SWS. Reduced metabolic demand during sleep cannot explain the diminished minute ventilation because partial pressure of arterial CO_2 ($PaCO_2$) increases during sleep (Krieger, 2000). It is possible that sleep-related neuronal mechanisms actively suppress ventilation, since minute ventilation decreases during sleep even in a hypercapnic environment. During SWS, airway resistance markedly increases due to decreased tonus of the upper airway muscles, whereas decreases in the contraction of intercostal muscles and of the diaphragm are small (Krieger, 2000). Therefore, sleep affects the neurons regulating the upper airway and those controlling the thorax in different manners.

Hypoxic and hypercapnic ventilatory responses are also vigilance-state dependent (QW > SWS > REM). The pulmonary stretch receptor reflex and irritant receptor reflex are also suppressed during sleep, and hence, cough develops only after arousal from sleep (Douglas, 2000). Although these phenomena are well known, the underlying mechanism remains to be elucidated.

Because basal respiration and respiratory reflex regulations are significantly different between the awake and sleep states and orexin regulates sleep/awake states, orexin may represent missing connection between the vigilance state and vigilance-state-dependent respiratory control (Figure 1). To test our hypothesis, we assessed the baseline characteristics of ventilation and the chemoreceptor reflex in response to hypoxia and hypercapnia during the sleep/awake periods, using our previously established method for the simultaneous measurements of vigilance states and ventilation in mice (Nakamura et al., 2003; Nakamura et al., 2004). In short, ventilation was recorded and a cortical electroencephalogram and a nuchal electromyogram were also obtained. Further, body movement was recorded in a specially designed flow-through whole-body plethysmographic chamber. The respiratory parameters during QW, SWS, and REM sleep were separately determined. The data during active wakefulness were not analyzed further because of contamination by artifacts originating from the animal's gross body movements.

2.1.1. Basal ventilation in orexin deficient mice

When the mice breathed normal room air, the respiratory frequency and tidal volume of the ORX-KO mice tended to be higher and lower, respectively, than those of the wild-type mice during both the awake and sleep periods. In other words, the ventilation in the ORX-KO mice tended to be shallow and fast. However, the minute ventilation was almost identical between the ORX-KO and the wild-type mice during every vigilance state (Figure 2) (Nakamura et al., 2007). For mice of both the genotypes, the respiratory frequency (QW > SWS, REM) and tidal volume (QW > SWS > REM) showed a clear sleep-wake dependency. Fragmentation of sleep episodes in the ORX-KO mice did not distort the relationship between vigilance states and minute ventilation (Nakamura et al., 2007). In addition, there was no difference in the circadian rhythm of ventilation (both with regard to cycle length and amplitude) (Kuwaki et al., 2005), although total sleep time was longer and movements were fewer in the ORX-KO mice during the night (Kuwaki et al., 2005). Therefore, orexin does not appear to contribute to basal breathing when the animal is at rest and under room air conditions.

2.1.2. Chemoreflex across vigilance states in orexin deficient mice

The magnitudes of the hypercapnic (5% CO_2–21% O_2 and 10% CO_2–21% O_2) and hypoxic (15% O_2) ventilatory responses in both the ORX-KO and wild-type mice showed a clear dependence on the vigilance state (Figure 2) (Nakamura et al., 2007). Namely, the order of the magnitude of changes in the minute ventilation was QW > SWS > REM, irrespective of the stimulus and genotypes (except for hypercapnic response in ORX-KO; QW ≈ SWS). In contrast to such a general similarity between the mutants and the controls, the hypercapnic responses in the ORX-KO mice during QW were significantly attenuated to approximately half the wild-type value when evaluated as an increase in the minute ventilation. When evaluated as the slope of the hypercapnic chemoreflex, the hypercapnic ventilatory response of the ORX-KO mice did not increase with arousal from sleep, although the SWS > REM relationship was preserved as in the wild-type mice (Figure 2, lower panel).

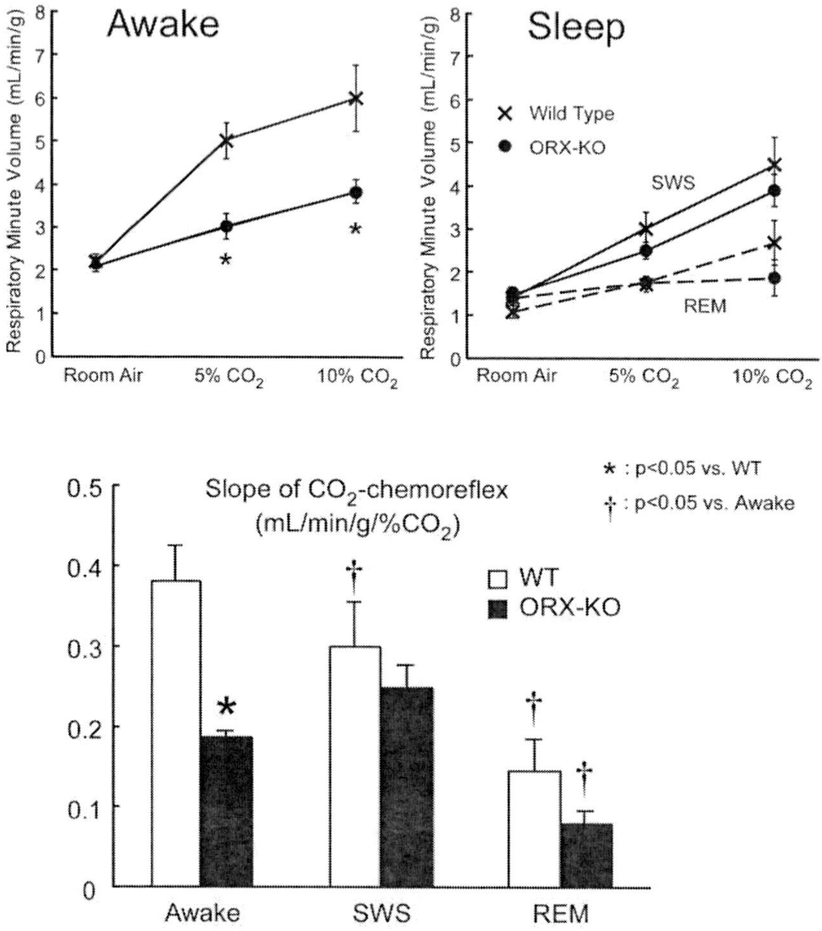

Figure 2. Hypercapnic responses of respiratory minute volume in wild-type (WT) mice and prepro-orexin knockout mice (ORX-KO) during quiet awake (upper left panel) and sleep (upper right panel) periods. (Lower panel) Hypercapnic responses are evaluated by calculating the slope of the relationship between inspired CO_2 concentration and respiratory minute volume. Data are presented as means ± SEM of 5 WT mice and 5 ORX-KO mice. Abbreviations: SWS, slow wave sleep; REM, rapid-eye-movement sleep. (Adapted from Nakamura et al., 2007).

On the other hand, there was no difference in the hypoxic ventilatory responses between the ORX-KO and the wild-type mice during QW and between the hypercapnic ventilatory responses during SWS and REM sleep. We cannot compare hypoxic ventilatory responses during sleep periods because the stimuli were insufficient to elicit any ventilatory response from either group of mice in this experimental setup (inhalation of 15% O_2). Nevertheless, we can say that the abnormal hypercapnic responses of the ORX-KO mice are vigilance-state dependent and not general occurrences.

To confirm whether the abovementioned respiratory abnormality in the ORX-KO mice is attributable orexin deficiency, we examined the possible effects of orexin supplementation in ORX-KO mice and that of the administration of the orexin receptor antagonist SB-334867 (Smart et al., 2001; Yamamoto et al., 2002) to wild-type mice. The drugs were intracerebroventricularly administered before a hypercapnic gas mixture was introduced in the body plethysmographic chamber. Because orexin-A and orexin-B have a strong wakefulness-promoting effect, we measured the chemoreflex only during the QW period. As expected, the supplementation with orexin-A or orexin-B (3 nmol) partially restored the hypercapnic chemoreflex in the ORX-KO mice (Figure 3) (Deng et al., 2007). The order of potency of orexin-A and -B differed between the awake-promoting effect (A > B) and respiratory effect (A ≤ B). Therefore, the respiratory effect of orexin appeared not secondary to its awake-promoting effect. In addition, injection of SB-334867 (30 nmol) to the wild-type mice decreased the hypercapnic chemoreflex without affecting the vigilance state (Figure 3). SB-334867 by itself did not affect basal ventilation, supporting our notion that orexin is not involved in the basal respiratory control at resting state. In line with our observation, Nattie's group recently reported that microdialysis of SB-334867 (5 mM) into the rats' retrotrapezoid nucleus reduced hypercapnic ventilatory response predominantly in wakefulness (Dias et al., 2009). Thus, retrotrapezoid nucleus seems at least one of the responsible sites for orexinergic modulation of hypercapnic chemostimulation. Orexinergic neurons *per se* seem to be also involved in hypercapnic activation of breathing because hypercapnia activates orexinergic neurons in vitro (Williams et al., 2007) and in vivo (Sunanaga et al., 2009).

There is an apparent inconsistency about receptor subtypes involved in ventilatory modulation by orexins. Orexin-B has a 10-fold selectivity for the orexin-2 receptor (Sakurai et al., 1998), thus the orexin-2 receptor appears to have played a larger part in the hypercapnic ventilatory response in the ORX-KO. On the other hand, blockade of the orexin-1 receptor by SB334867 (over 100-fold selective to the orexin-1 receptor at least in vitro) weakened hypercapnic chemoreflex of the wild-type mice, indicating that the orexin-1 receptor is necessary for chemoreflex control. Although we have not tested a blocker for the orexin-2 receptor, it is likely to weaken hypercapnic chemoreflex to a larger degree than SB334867.

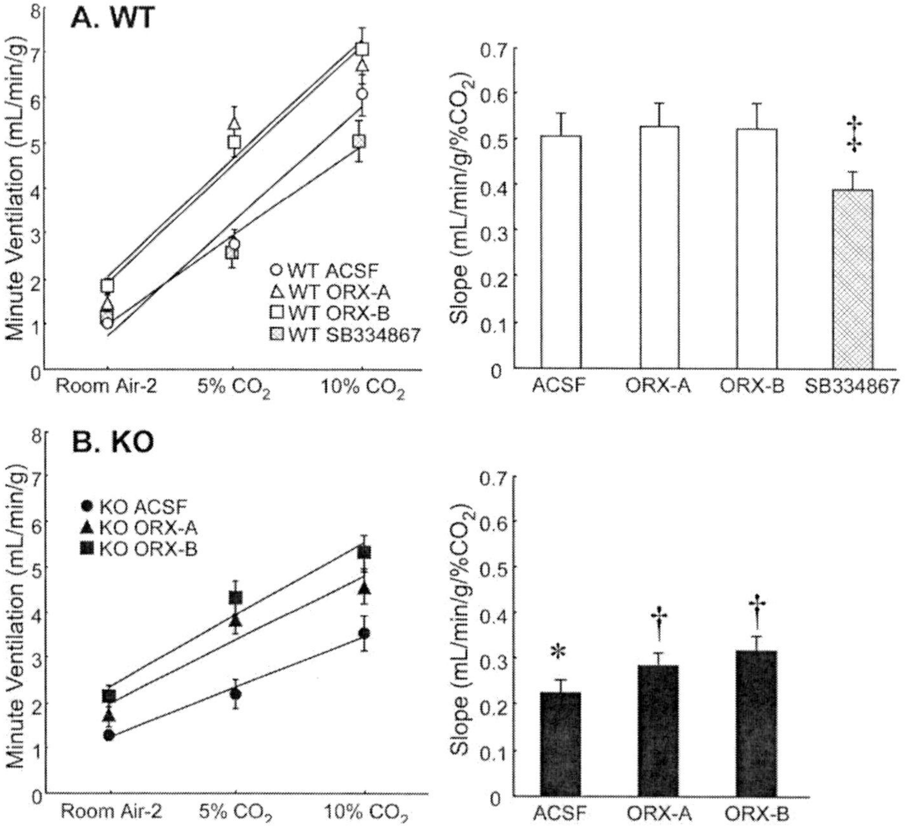

Figure 3. Hypercapnic responses of minute ventilation during quiet wakefulness. Absolute values of minute ventilation are plotted against the inspired CO_2 concentrations in the left panel, and slopes calculated by linear regression analysis are shown in the right panel. Wild-type mice (WT; n = 6-7, A) and prepro-orexin knockout mice (KO; n = 9, B) received artificial cerebrospinal fluid (ACSF, 2 µl), orexin-A (ORX-A, 3 nmol), orexin-B (ORX-B, 3 nmol), or the orexin receptor antagonist SB334667 (30 nmol). Data are presented as means ± SEM. * $P < 0.05$ compared with ACSF-treated WT in A. † $P < 0.05$ compared with ACSF-treated KO. ‡ $P < 0.05$ compared with ACSF- and vehicle-treated WT. (Adapted from Deng et al. 2007).

Based on these results, we have proposed that the hypercapnic response during sleep periods relies on unknown mechanisms that are independent of orexin, and the response is augmented by orexin during awake periods. This proposal is consistent with reports stating that the spontaneous activity of orexin-containing neurons is increased during awake periods and is decreased during sleep periods (Lee et al., 2005; Mileykovskiy et al., 2005). In addition, CO_2 activated the orexinergic neurons in hypothalamic slice preparations (Williams et al., 2007) and in mice in vivo (Sunanaga et al., 2009). On the other hand, wakefulness drive to breathing has been proposed to increase hypercapnic responsiveness (Phillipson, 1978), and the administration of orexin may increase ventilation via its awakening effect. However, our results for knockout mice clearly demonstrated that waking *per se* could not augment the hypercapnic responsiveness in the absence of orexin.

2.1.3. Breathing regulation during sleep in orexin deficient mice

In ORX-KO mice, the qualitative characteristics of sleep apneas, defined as cessation of ventilation for at least 2 respiratory cycles, were similar to those observed in the wild-type mice (Nakamura et al., 2003; Nakamura et al., 2004). Namely, spontaneous and post-sigh apneas were observed during SWS, and spontaneous but not post-sigh apneas were observed during REM sleep, although sighs were recorded during not only SWS but also REM sleep (Nakamura et al., 2007). Moreover, all the apneas appeared to be of central origin because the intercostal EMG indicated that firing stopped during the apneic episodes. From a quantitative point of view, however, spontaneous apneas during both SWS and REM sleep were significantly more frequent (about 2–3 times higher) in the ORX-KO mice than in the wild-type mice (Figure 4), whereas the frequency of post-sigh apneas during SWS did not differ between the two. Such differences were preserved when the breathing gas mixture was changed to hypoxic or hypercapnic gases. We have recently found more severe sleep apnea in ORX/ATX-Tg mice (black column in Figure 4; Y. Tagaito and T. Kuwaki, unpublished observation).

These results indicate that orexin exerts an inhibitory effect on the genesis of spontaneous sleep apneas. Our observation is similar to a previous finding that indicates a high incidence of sleep apneas among narcolepsy patients (Chokroverty, 1986). Thus, orexin appears to be indispensable not only during wakefulness (refer to section 2.1.2.) but also during sleep periods for respiratory integrity; this is despite the fact that orexin's roles in respiratory regulation differ between vigilance states. This proposal may appear to be in conflict with reports stating that the spontaneous activity of orexin-containing neurons increases during awake periods and is decreased during sleep periods (Lee et al., 2005; Mileykovskiy et al., 2005). However, these reports also stated small but considerable increases in orexinergic neuronal activity during the REM period that were higher than those recorded during the SWS period. Isolated orexin neurons that are deprived of any synaptic input show spontaneous activity (Yamanaka et al., 2003), indicating their potential firing during sleep. The magnitude of exaggeration of spontaneous sleep apnea by orexin deficiency was greater during REM sleep than during SWS (Nakamura et al., 2007). Thus, the activation of orexinergic neurons during REM sleep may exert an inhibitory effect on the genesis of spontaneous sleep apneas. In addition, functional dichotomy in orexin-containing neurons has been suggested; orexin neurons in the LHA regulate reward processing for both food and abused drugs, whereas those in the PFA and DMH regulate arousal from sleep and the response to stress (Harris et al., 2006). Therefore, it may be possible that a subset of orexinergic neurons contributes to CO_2 sensitivity during awake periods and another subset contributes to the inhibition of spontaneous apnea during sleep.

We do not consider that the decreased influence of orexin can explain all human sleep apneas because most human apneas that are reported are of the obstructive type. Nevertheless, there are good reasons to suspect the possible involvement of orexin deficiency in some cases of human apneas, most probably in narcoleptic patients. First, orexin neurons are activated by hypoglycemia (Cai et al., 2001) and are inhibited by glucose (Yamanaka et al., 2003; Burdakov et al., 2005) through the TWIK-related acid-sensitive K^+ (TASK) subfamily of tandem-pore potassium channels (Burdakov et al., 2006). Hyperglycemia is a powerful predictor of impaired breathing during sleep in both humans and animals (Polotsky et al., 2001; Punjabi et al., 2004). Second, orexin innervates the hypoglossal nucleus (Fung et al., 2001) that plays a major role in preventing obstructive sleep apnea (Jordan et al., 2008). Third, some obstructive sleep apnea patients showed low levels of plasma orexin (Busquets et al., 2004; Sakurai et al., 2005a), although a contradictory result (Igarashi et al., 2003) and no change in CSF orexin (Kanbayashi et al., 2003) have also been reported. Finally, at least during the induction phase of sleep, most apneas are thought to be of central origin in humans (Krieger, 2000). As mentioned in section 1.1., narcolepsy patients had frequent sleep apneas and they were thought to be central in type (Chokroverty, 1986).

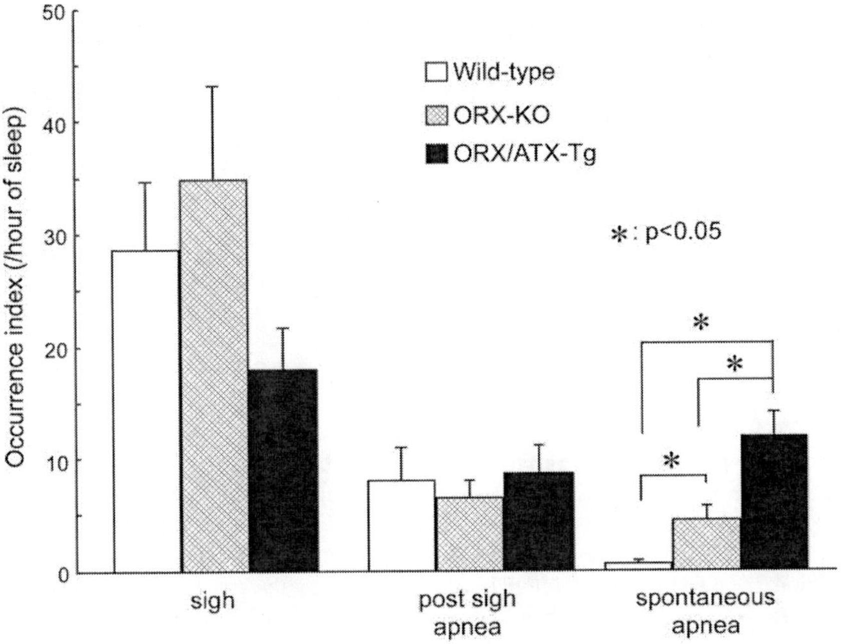

Figure 4. Sigh and apnea occurrence index in wild-type mice, prepro-orexin knockout mice (ORX-KO), and orexin neuron-ablated mice (ORX/ATX-Tg) during sleep when the animals breathed room air. Data are presented as means ± SEM of wild-type mice (open bar, n = 5), ORX-KO mice (hatched bar, n = 5), and ORX/ATX-Tg mice (solid bar, n = 6). (Data for wild-type and ORX-KO mice are adapted from Nakamura et al. (2007). Data for ORX/ATX-Tg mice are unpublished observation by Y. Tagaito & T. Kuwaki).

Repetitive intermittent hypoxia, a model of sleep apnea-induced hypoxemia, induces long-lasting (> 1h) augmentation of respiratory motor output that occurs even after the cessation of hypoxic stimuli (Powell et al., 1998; Feldman et al., 2003; Mitchell et al., 2003). This phenomenon is called as respiratory long-term facilitation (LTF). LTF relies on serotonin-containing neurons in the raphe nuclei and is pattern sensitive, i.e., it occurs after repetitive (>3 times) intermittent hypoxia but not after sustained hypoxia (Millhorn et al., 1980; Feldman et al., 2003). We hypothesized a possible contribution of orexin to LTF because the raphe nuclei receive dense projections from the orexin-containing neurons in the hypothalamus (Peyron et al., 1998; Nambu et al., 1999; Berthoud et al., 2005) and the pattern-sensitive nature of LTF resembles the behavioral state-dependent nature of the orexinergic control of respiration.

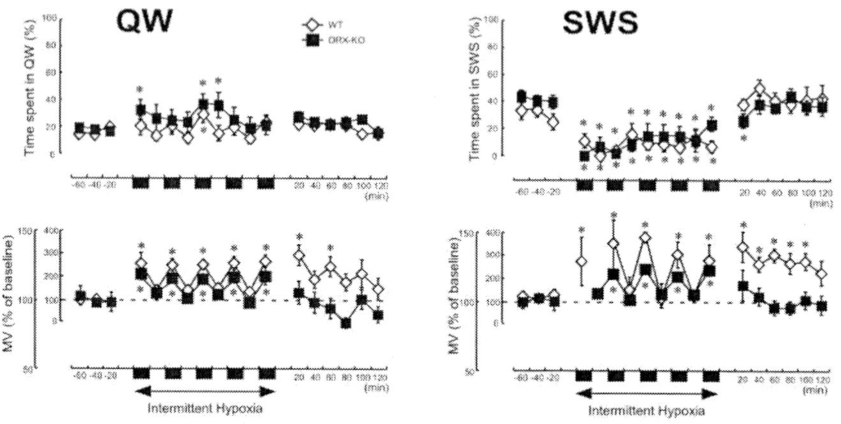

Figure 5. Time-related changes in vigilance state and minute ventilation before, during, and after intermittent hypoxia. Upper panels: Time spent in quiet wakefulness (QW) and slow-wave sleep (SWS). Wild-type mice (WT, open symbols, n = 8) and prepro-orexin knockout mice (ORX-KO, closed symbols, n = 8) received intermittent hypoxic stimulation; the duration of the stimulation is indicated by the arrow. The black bar under the abscissa indicates the time when hypoxic gas (10% CO_2) was introduced into the plethysmographic chamber. Lower panels: Long-term responses to hypoxia. Changes in minute ventilation (MV) as a percentage of baseline values (pre-hypoxia = 100%) were averaged every 20 min (before and after the stimulation, the scale range is 50–150%) or every 5 min (during stimulation, the scale range is 0–400%). MV was separately calculated for QW (left) and SWS (right). Ventilatory data for the first hypoxic challenge (ORX-KO) and the subsequent room air period (WT) are missing because no animal showed SWS. Note that 2 scale ranges are used to show time-related changes at a higher resolution. Data are presented as means ± SEM. * $P < 0.05$ compared with the baseline value. (Adapted from Terada et al. 2008).

To test our hypothesis, we measured the ventilation in freely-moving ORX-KO and wild-type littermates before, during, and after exposure to intermittent hypoxia (5 times of 5-min 10% O_2), sustained hypoxia (25-min 10% O_2), or sham stimulation (Terada et al., 2008). The acute hypoxic response observed during intermittent hypoxia and sustained hypoxia exposure was not different between the mice of the 2 genotypes, as was the case in the experiment stated in the section 2.1.2. Following intermittent hypoxia exposure, although the wild-type littermates showed augmented minute ventilation (Figure 5, by 20.0 ± 4.5% during QW and 26.5 ± 5.3% during SWS) for 2 h, the ORX-KO littermates showed no significant increase (by –3.1 ± 4.6% during QW and 0.3 ± 5.2% during SWS). Both genotypes showed no LTF after sustained hypoxia or sham stimulation.

These results indicate that orexin is needed to elicit LTF during both awake and sleep periods. In other words, the role of orexin in LTF appears to be vigilance-state independent. However, it is important to point out that repetitive hypoxic stimulation awakens the animals (Figure 5), similar to the effect of sleep apneas on humans (Bassiri et al., 2000). Thus, it is possible that hypoxia activates orexinergic neurons, and activated orexinergic neurons in turn induce arousal from sleep (or a trend toward arousal from sleep; "micro arousal") and subsequent LTF. Indeed, orexinergic neurons receive innervations from the nucleus tractus solitarius (Sakurai et al., 2005b) where the first-order relay neurons for hypoxic information are located. Moreover, “micro arousal” depends on orexin as is evidenced by a lack of increase in the ß-band power of the electroencephalogram upon providing stimulation to the hypothalamus in the ORX-KO mice (Kayaba et al., 2003). There is some evidence indicating that the administration of orexin increases ventilation during both the awake (Deng et al., 2007) and anesthetized (and presumably during sleep) (Young et al., 2005; Zhang et al., 2005) states. Although the abovementioned statements are hypothetical, whether or not hypoxia activates orexin-containing neurons in the hypothalamus remains debatable. This is despite the fact that hypoxia activates some neurons in the hypothalamus (Berquin et al., 2000) and hypercapnia activates orexinergic neurons (Williams et al., 2007; Sunanaga et al., 2009). Nevertheless, it can be said that the probable role of orexin in respiratory modulation is “state”-dependent, such that “state” includes not only vigilance states but also stimulus-triggered states. This notion is supported by our observation that orexin is indispensable to stress-induced cardiorespiratory augmentation (section 2.2.) (Kayaba et al., 2003; Zhang et al., 2006a; Zhang et al., 2006b; Kuwaki, 2008; Kuwaki et al., 2008).

2.2. Cardiorespiratory Regulation during Stress

Research on neural mechanisms of state-dependent adjustments of central autonomic regulation have been sparse, despite its importance from the perspective of quality-of-life. Our daily life does not only involve calm, resting states. Life is full of perturbations that induce active conditions, such as movements, eating, and communicating. During such active periods, cardiorespiratory regulation must be adjusted for bodily demands, which differ from those during resting states, by modulating or resetting homeostatic points (Kumada et al., 1990). Localization of orexinergic cell bodies in PFA and DMH prompted us to examine possible role of orexin in the defense response against stressors because stimulation to them elicited behavioral "rage" along with the specific autonomic responses that was termed the "defense response" (Figure 6) (Hess, 1954; Jordan, 1990; DiMicco et al., 2002).

Animals cope with stressors by two strategies. An active coping strategy (fight or flight) is evoked if the stress is predictable, controllable, or escapable. A passive coping strategy (immobility or decreased responsiveness to the environment) is evoked if the stress is inescapable. The active strategy is associated with sympathoexcitation (hypertension, tachycardia), whereas the passive strategy is associated with sympathoinhibition and/or parasympathetic activation (hypotension, bradycardia). The passive strategy also helps to facilitate recovery and healing. The active strategy is also called the "fight or flight response" from a behavioral point of view or "defense response" from an autonomic point of view. The passive strategy is sometimes called "playing dead" or "paradoxical fear". Distinct neural substrates mediating active vs. passive emotional coping have been identified within the brainstem (Nosaka, 1996; Bandler et al., 2000).

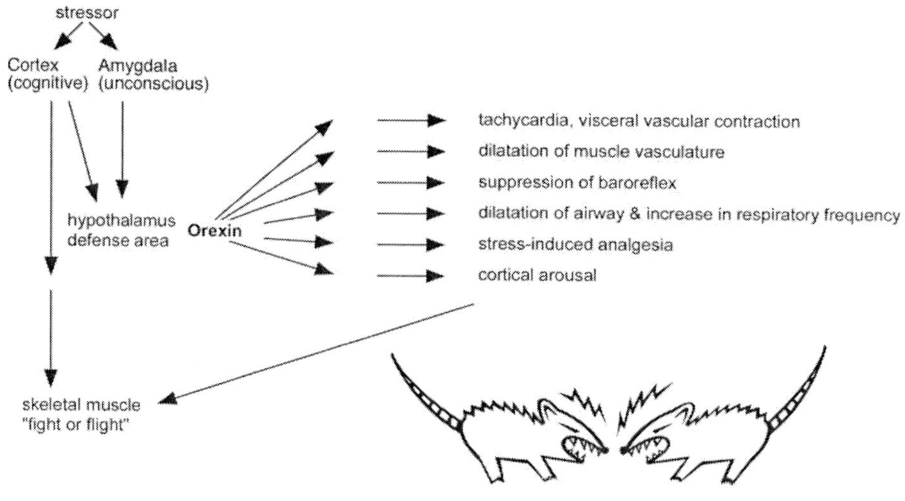

Figure 6. Multi facet nature of the defense response. Simultaneous and coordinated changes in the cardiorespiratory, sensory, and thermoregulatory systems supports the efficiency of the behavioral response of fight or flight. Orexin play a role as a master switch of these orchestrated responses.

Several neurotransmitters have been proposed to be involved in modulation of the efferent pathways of defense responses against stressors. For example, activation of serotonin (5HT)-1A receptors in the medullary raphe reduces cardiovascular changes (Nalivaiko et al., 2005), and inhibition of 5HT-3 receptors in the nucleus tractus solitarius prevents the baroreflex bradycardia inhibition during the defense response (Sévoz-Couche et al., 2003). Microinjections of adenosine into the rostral ventrolateral medulla augment the increase in blood pressure evoked by electrical stimulation of the hypothalamic defense area (Thomas et al., 1996). The pros and cons of glutamate participation in the cardiovascular component of the defense response have been debated (Sun et al., 1986; Kiely et al., 1994). However, to date, there is no report on the molecular basis of the defense response underlying the multi-facet nature of simultaneous and coordinated changes in the cardiovascular, respiratory, sensory, and behavioral parameters.

We hypothesized that intrinsic orexin, synthesized in the PFA/DMH, regulates the multi-faceted features of the defense response (Figure 6). In fact, stressors activate orexinergic neurons (Ida et al., 2000; Zhu et al., 2002; Espana et al., 2003; Winsky-Sommerer et al., 2004; Watanabe et al., 2005; Kuwaki et al., 2007). Anatomical (section 1.4) and pharmacological (section 3.1) evidence support our hypothesis. To examine our hypothesis, we used ORX-KO and ORX/ATX-Tg mice and observed their responses to direct stimulation to the hypothalamus and natural stressful stimuli. Measured changes include blood pressure, heart rate, muscular blood flow, respiratory frequency and tidal volume, and suppression of the baroreceptor reflex and pain sensitivity.

2.2.1. Basal cardiorespiratory parameters in orexin deficient mice

We found that basal blood pressure in ORX-KO and ORX/ATX-Tg mice was significantly lower by about 20 mmHg in both anesthetized and conscious conditions (Kayaba et al., 2003; Zhang et al., 2006a). Circadian fluctuation of blood pressure and heart rate was similar between ORX-KO and wild-type mice except that blood pressure in ORX-KO mice was consistently lower during both dark phase and light phase. Drowsiness and lower activity in ORX-KO cannot explain the difference in blood pressure because these behavioral abnormalities were only apparent during dark phase (active phase for nocturnal mice) while lower blood pressure was observed even in the light phase when the behavioral abnormalities were not significant. Alpha-adrenergic blockade with prazosin or ganglion blockade with hexamethonium cancelled the difference in basal blood pressure. Heart rate and cardiac contractile parameters by echocardiography did not differ from those in wild-type mice. These results indicate lower sympathetic vasoconstrictor tone in orexin deficient mice. As described in the section 2.1.1., basal ventilation (respiratory frequency and tidal volume) was not significantly altered in ORX-KO mice nor ORX/ATX-Tg mice.

2.2.2. Cardiorespiratory parameters during stress in orexin deficient mice

To date, we have five lines of evidence that support our hypothesis of possible contribution of orexin to the defense response. First, stimulation of the PFA with the GABA-A receptor antagonist, bicuculline, attenuated the defense response in urethane-anesthetized ORX-KO and ORX/ATX-Tg mice. Increases in arterial blood pressure, heart rate, respiratory frequency, and ß-band power of the electroencephalogram (an index of cortical arousal) were smaller and/or shorter lasting in ORX-KO than in the wild-type littermates (Kayaba et al., 2003). In a similar manner, increased blood pressure, heart rate, and respiratory minute volume and vascular dilatation in the skeletal muscle were attenuated in the ORX/ATX-Tg mice (Figure 7) (Zhang et al., 2006a).

Secondly, suppression of the baroreceptor reflex during the defense response was attenuated in the ORX/ATX-Tg mice, whereas characteristics of the baroreceptor reflex (gain and slope) at rest were normal in these mice (Zhang et al., 2006a). During the defense response, the baroreceptor reflex is suppressed or reset to a higher pressure range to allow an blood pressure greater than that in the resting condition. Orexin appeared to contribute to the suppression of the baroreflex during the defense response, but not to the baroreflex during the resting condition.

Third, an attenuation of the defense response in the ORX-KO and ORX/ATX-Tg mice was also observed by natural stimulation in unanesthetized and freely moving conditions (Figure 8). We tested the defense response in conscious animals using the resident-intruder test or air-jet stress paradigm to exclude the possibility of the observed difference between the orexin-deficient mice and the wild-type littermates resulting from differences in anesthetic susceptibilities. As expected, the emotional stressor-induced increases in the blood pressure, heart rate, and locomotor activity were smaller in orexin-deficient mice (ORX-KO and ORX/ATX-Tg) than those in the wild-type littermates (Kayaba et al., 2003; Zhang et al., 2006a).

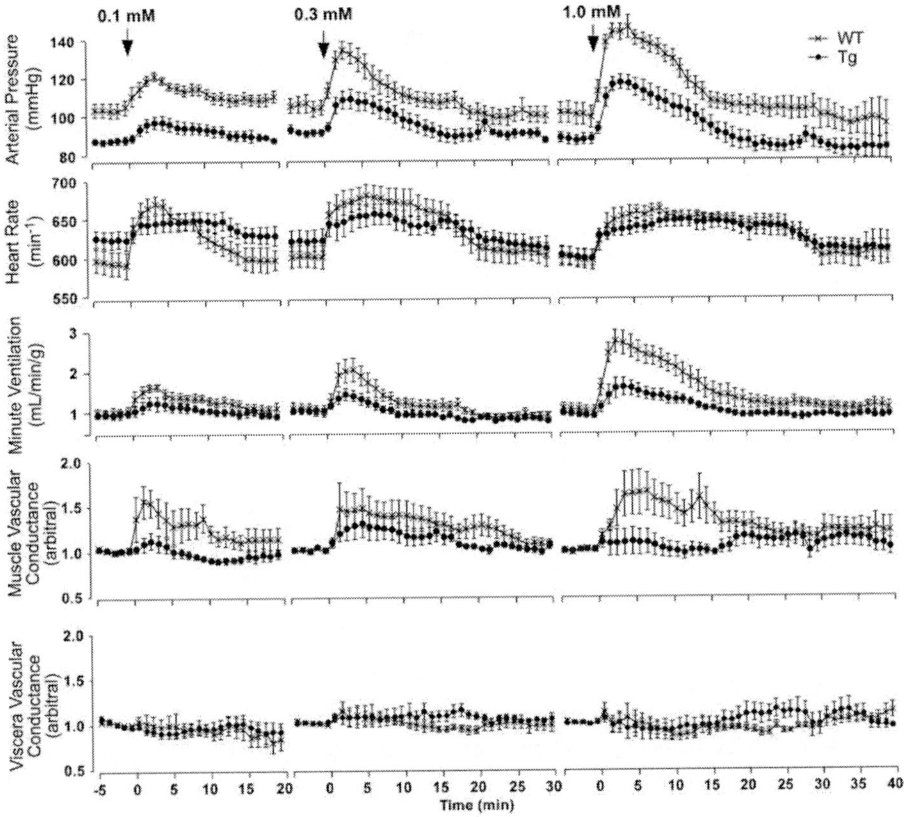

Figure 7. Effects of microinjection of bicuculline methiodide to the perifornical area in wild-type (WT) mice and orexin/ataxin-3 transgenic mice (Tg) on arterial blood pressure, heart rate, respiratory minute ventilation, and the muscular and the visceral vascular conductance. Arrowheads indicate timing of microinjection of bicuculline (20 nl). Data are presented as mean ± SEM of 8 WT mice and 9 Tg mice. (Adapted from Zhang et al. 2006a).

Fourth, foot shock stress-induced analgesia was attenuated in the ORX-KO mice. In wild-type mice, the foot shock induced long-lasting analgesia, as evidenced by increases in the tail flick latency from noxious hot water. Although ORX-KO mice showed moderate analgesia, that effect was significantly smaller than that shown by the wild-type littermates (Watanabe et al., 2005). In line with this result, we observed numerous expressions of c-fos, a marker for cellular activation, in neurons with orexin-like immunoreactivity after foot shock (Watanabe et al., 2005; Kuwaki et al., 2007).

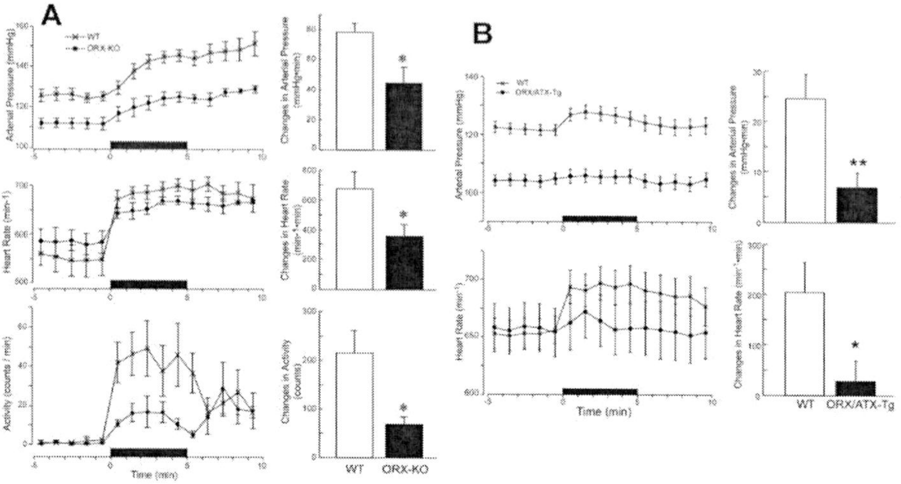

Figure 8. Cardiovascular and behavioral responses during natural stressful stimulation in conscious orexin deficient mice and their wild-type (WT) littermates. (A) Resident-intruder test was performed in radio telemeter-indwelled freely moving wild-type (WT) and orexin knockout (ORX-KO) mice. The presence of an intruder is indicated by the horizontal solid bar. Right side panels are the changes in blood pressure, heart rate, and activity expressed as area under the curve (AUC) during five minutes when an intruder was present in the same cage. (B) Air jet stress was applied to catheter-indwelling lightly restrained WT and orexin/ataxin-3 transgenic (ORX/ATX-Tg) mice. Duration of air jet stress is indicated by the horizontal solid bar. Right side panels are the changes in arterial pressure and heart rate expressed as AUC during 5 min of the stress. Data are presented as means ± SEM of 6-8 mice in each genotype. * $p<0.05$, ** $p<0.01$ vs. WT mice. (Adapted from Kayaba et al. 2003; Zhang et al. 2006a).

Fifth, disinhibition of the amygdala or the BNST by an injection of bicuculline in urethane-anesthetized ORX/ATX-Tg mice scarcely caused cardiorespiratory activation that were consistently observed in wild-type control mice (Figure 9) (Zhang et al., 2009).

From these results, we concluded that orexin-containing neurons in the PFA/DMH mediate at least a part of amygdala- and BNST-induced cardiorespiratory responses and act as a master switch to activate multiple efferent pathways of the defense response. Orexin, but not its co-transmitters in the neurons, appeared to be important, at least for changes in blood pressure, heart rate, and respiration (Zhang et al., 2006b).

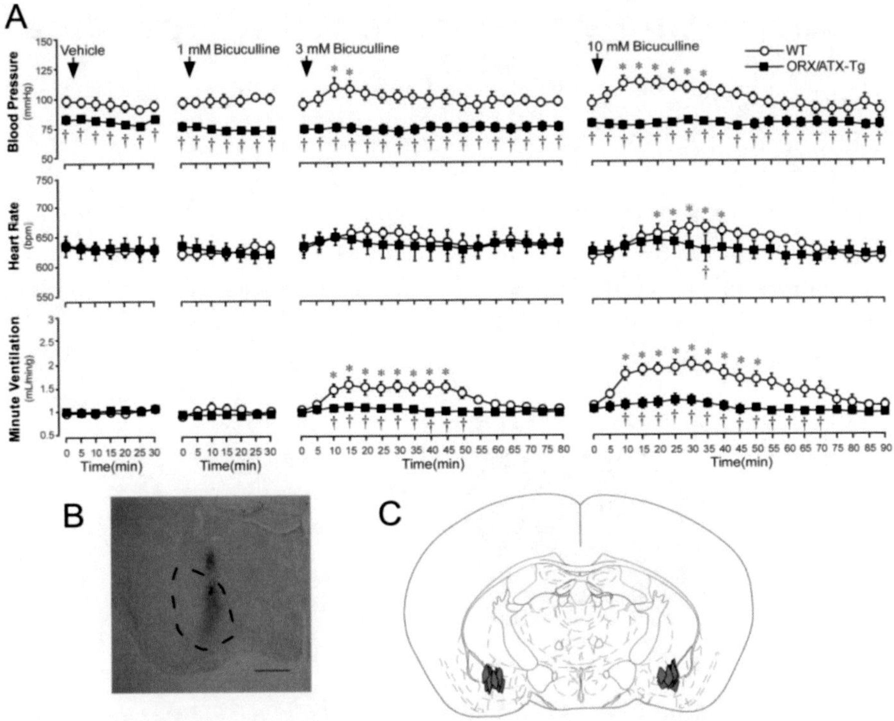

Figure 9. Effects on blood pressure, heart rate, and minute ventilation of microinjecting vehicle and bicuculline methiodide into the amygdala in wild-type (WT) mice and orexin neuron-ablated (ORX/ATX-Tg) mice. (A) Time course of the responses. Arrowheads indicate timing of microinjection of bicuculline (20nl). * $P < 0.05$ vs. time 0 (repeated measure ANOVA followed by post hoc test of Dunnett); † $P<0.05$ vs. WT mice (unpaired two-tailed t-test). (B) Typical photograph showing injection site as evaluated by distribution of the same volume of Evans blue dye. Dashed line indicates border of the amygdala. Scale bar = 1mm. (C) Summary for injection sites. Left side shows dye-distribution in WT mice and right side shows that in ORX/ATX-Tg mice. In the actual experiment, drugs and dye were injected into unilateral amygdala. Data are presented as mean ± SEM of 8 WT mice and 8 ORX/ATX-Tg mice. (Adapted from Zhang et al. 2009).

3. Supporting Evidence in Wild-Type Mice and Rats

3.1. Exogenous Administration of Orexin

The exogenous administration of orexin induces analgesia (Yamamoto et al., 2002), cardiovascular (Samson et al., 1999; Shirasaka et al., 1999; Chen et al., 2000; Antunes et al., 2001; Machado et al., 2002; Zhang et al., 2005), and respiratory (Young et al., 2005; Zhang et al., 2005; Deng et al., 2007; Dutschmann et al., 2007) activation.

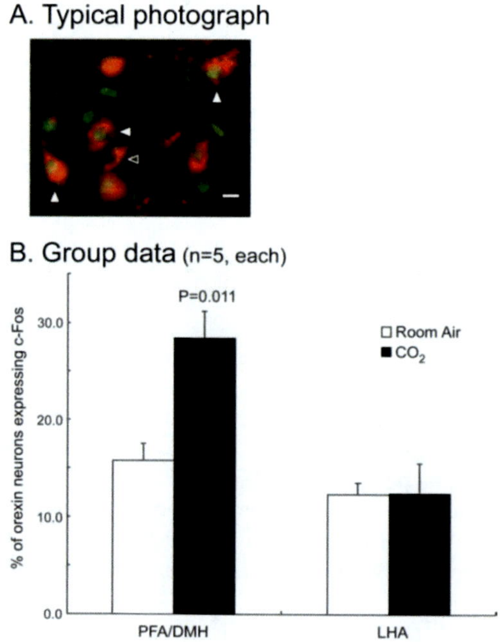

Figure 10. Effect of CO_2- or room air-breathing on c-Fos expression in the orexinergic neurons. (A) Representative photographs of double immunostaining for orexin and c-Fos, a marker of neuronal activation, in the hypothalamus of mice. Brains were sampled after 3 hours inhalation of hypercapnic gas mixture (10% CO_2, 21% O_2, and residual N_2). Orexin was stained in red and c-Fos was stained in green. Yellow designates cells stained for both orexin and c-Fos. Filled triangles indicate double stained cells and open triangles indicate orexin-containing but not c-Fos expressing cells. Scale bar = 10 μm. (B) Percent of orexin-immunopositive cells that are expressing c-Fos. Abbreviations: PFA, perifornical area; DMH, dorsomedial hypothalamus; LHA, lateral hypothalamic area. (Adapted from Sunanaga et al. 2009).

3.2. Functional Neuroanatomy

We found that inhalation of gas mixture of 10% CO_2, 21% O_2, and residual N_2 to awake and freely moving wild-type mice for 3 hours significantly increased expression of c-Fos, a marker for cellular activation, in the orexin-containing cells that were located in the PFA/DMH (15.8±1.6% for room air vs. 28.4±2.7% for CO_2, p=0.011) but not in the LHA (12.3±1.2% for room air vs. 12.4±3.0% for CO_2) (Figure 10) (Sunanaga et al., 2009). Although this methodology cannot differentiate between direct effect of CO_2 on the orexin-containing neurons and indirect one through other neurons, inhalation of CO_2 did activate the orexin-containing neurons in vivo.

We also observed numerous expressions of c-Fos in neurons with orexin-like immunoreactivity after foot shock stress (Watanabe et al., 2005; Kuwaki et al., 2007). Moreover, disinhibition of the amygdala or BNST induced significantly larger numbers of orexin positive neurons that expressed c-Fos in the PFA/DMH (58.2±6.4 % into the amygdala and 66.4±6.6 % into BNST) than did vehicle (18.2±4.4 % into the amygdala and 28.3±2.1 % into BNST). Disinhibition to the BNST induced widespread expression of c-Fos not only in orexin-containing neurons but also other neurons in the hypothalamus (Zhang et al., 2009).

These results are well coincide with observed autonomic malfunctions in ORX-KO and ORX/ATX-Tg mice.

4. Conclusion

Here, we summarized autonomic malfunctions in mice model of narcolepsy. Orexin probably contributes to the waking-associated augmentation of the hypercapnic chemoreflex, suppression of sleep apnea, repetitive intermittent hypoxia-induced ventilatory LTF, determination of basal sympathetic nerve activity and blood pressure, simultaneous activation of multiple efferent pathways of the defense response. Although these responses may appear to be independent, we assume that the common feature of the responses is a state-dependent adjustment of central autonomic regulation. Based on these results, and other suggested functions of orexin neurons and their anatomical connections (Willie et al., 2001; Saper et al., 2005; Sakurai, 2007), we propose orexin-related central neural pathways that subserve emotional and state-dependent modifications of cardiorespiratory homeostatic reflexes, as shown in Figure 1.

Diversity in the synaptic control of cardiovascular and respiratory neurons appears to be necessary for animals to adapt themselves to constantly changing situations and behavioral states. The orexin system is likely to function as one of the essential modulators for orchestrating the circuits that control autonomic functions and behavior. Deficiency of orexin induces not only narcolepsy but also diverse autonomic malfunctions.

Acknowledgments

Part of the study was supported by a Grant-in-Aid for Scientific Research (17590183, 18590203, 20590226) from the Ministry of Education, Culture, Sports, Science and Technology, Japan.

References

Abrahamson, E. E., Leak, R. K. & Moore, R. Y. (2001). The suprachiasmatic nucleus projects to posterior hypothalamic arousal systems. *Neuroreport*, *12*, 435-440.

Antunes, V. R., Brailoiu, G. C., Kwok, E. H., Scruggs, P. & Dun, N. J. (2001). Orexins/hypocretins excite rat sympathetic preganglionic neurons in vivo and in vitro. *Am. J. Physiol. Regul. Integr. Comp. Physiol.*, *281*, R1801-R1807.

Baker, T., Guilleminault, C., Nino-Murcia, G. & Dement, W. (1986). Comparative polysomnographic study of narcolepsy and idiopathic central nervous system hypersomnia. *Sleep*, *9*, 232-242.

Bandler, R., Keay, K. A., Floyd, N. & Price, J. (2000). Central circuits mediating patterned autonomic activity during active vs. passive emotional coping. *Brain Res. Bull.*, *53*, 95-104.

Bassiri, A. G. & Guilleminault, C. Clinical features and evaluation of obstructive sleep apnea-hypopnea syndrome. In: Kryger, MH, Roth, T & Dement, WC (Eds.) (2000). *Principles and Practice of Sleep Medicine*. Philadelphia: W.B. Saunders, 869-878.

Berquin, P., Bodineau, L., Gros, F. & Larnicol, N. (2000). Brainstem and hypothalamic areas involved in respiratory chemoreflexes: a Fos study in adult rats. *Brain Res.*, *857*, 30-40.

Berthoud, H. R., Patterson, L. M., Sutton, G. M., Morrison, C. & Zheng, H. (2005). Orexin inputs to caudal raphe neurons involved in thermal, cardiovascular, and gastrointestinal regulation. *Histochem. Cell Biol.*, *123*, 147-156.

Burdakov, D., Gerasimenko, O. & Verkhratsky, A. (2005). Physiological changes in glucose differentially modulate the excitability of hypothalamic melanin-concentrating hormone and orexin neurons in situ. *J. Neurosci.*, *25*, 2429-2433.

Burdakov, D., Jensen, L. T., Alexopoulos, H., Williams, R. H., Fearon, I. M., O'Kelly, I., Gerasimenko, O., Fugger, L. & Verkhratsky, A. (2006). Tandem-pore K+ channels mediate inhibition of orexin neurons by glucose. *Neuron*, *50*, 711-722.

Busquets, X., Barbe, F., Barcelo, A., de la Pena, M., Sigritz, N., Mayoralas, L., Ladaria, A. & Agusti, A. (2004). Decreased plasma levels of orexin-A in sleep apnea. *Respiration*, *71*, 575-579.

Cai, X. J., Evans, M. L., Lister, C. A., Leslie, R. A., Arch, J. R. S., Wilson, S. & Williams, G. (2001). Hypoglycemia activates orexin neurons and selectively increases hypothalamic orexin-B levels: Responses inhibited by feeding and possibly mediated by the nucleus of the solitary tract. *Diabetes*, *50*, 105-112.

Chemelli, R. M., Willie, J. T., Sinton, C. M., Elmquist, J. K., Scammell, T. E., Lee, C., Richardson, J. A., Williams, S. C., Xiong, Y., Kisanuki, Y., Fitch, T. E., Nakazato, M., Hammer, R. E., Saper, C. B. & Yanagisawa, M. (1999). Narcolepsy in orexin knockout mice: molecular genetics of sleep regulation. *Cell*, *98*, 437-451.

Chen, C. T., Hwang, L. L., Chang, J. K. & Dun, N. J. (2000). Pressor effects of orexins injected intracisternally and to rostral ventrolateral medulla of anesthetized rats. *Am. J. Physiol. Regul. Integr. Comp. Physiol.*, *278*, R692-R697.

Cheng, S. B., Kuchiiwa, S., Gao, H. Z., Kuchiiwa, T. & Nakagawa, S. (2003). Morphological study of orexin neurons in the hypothalamus of the Long-Evans rat, with special reference to co-expression of orexin and NADPH-diaphorase or nitric oxide synthase activities. *Neurosci. Res.*, *46*, 53-62.

Chokroverty, S. (1986). Sleep apnea in narcolepsy. *Sleep*, *9*, 250-253.

Chou, T. C., Lee, C. E., Lu, J., Elmquist, J. K., Hara, J., Willie, J. T., Beuckmann, C. T., Chemelli, R. M., Sakurai, T., Yanagisawa, M., Saper, C. B. & Scammell, T. E. (2001). Orexin (hypocretin) neurons contain dynorphin. *J. Neurosci.*, *21*, RC168,161-166.

de Lecea, L., Kilduff, T., Peyron, C., Gao, X., Foye, P., Danielson, P., Fukuhara, C., Battenberg, E., Gautvik, V., Bartlett, F. n., Frankel, W., van den Pol, A., Bloom, F., Gautvik, K. & Sutcliffe, J. (1998). The hypocretins: hypothalamus-specific peptides with neuroexcitatory activity. *Proc. Natl. Acad. Sci.*, USA., *95*, 322-327.

Deng, B.-S., Nakamura, A., Zhang, W., Yanagisawa, M., Fukuda, Y. & Kuwaki, T. (2007). Contribution of orexin in hypercapnic chemoreflex: Evidence from genetic and pharmacological disruption and supplementation studies in mice. *J. Appl. Physiol.*, *103*, 1772-1779.

Dergacheva, O., Wang, X., Huang, Z. G., Bouairi, E., Stephens, C., Gorini, C. & Mendelowitz, D. (2005). Hypocretin-1 (orexin-a) facilitates inhibitory and diminishes excitatory synaptic pathways to cardiac vagal neurons in the nucleus ambiguus. *J. Pharmacol. Exp. Ther.*, *314*, 1322-1327.

Dias, M., Li, A. & Nattie, E. (2009). Antagonism of orexin receptor-1 in the retrotrapezoid nucleus inhibits the ventilatory response to hypercapnia predominantly in wakefulness. *J. Physiol.*, *587*, 2059-2067.

DiMicco, J. A., Samuels, B. C., Zaretskaia, M. V. & Zaretsky, D. V. (2002). The dorsomedial hypothalamus and the response to stress: part renaissance, part revolution. *Pharmacol. Biochem. Behav.*, *71*, 469-480.

Douglas, N. J. Respiratory physiology: Control of ventilation. In: Kryger, MH, Roth, T & Dement, WC (Eds.) (2000). *Principles and Practice of Sleep Medicine*. Philadelphia: W.B. Saunders, 221-228.

Dun, N. J., Le Dun, S., Chen, C. T., Hwang, L. L., Kwok, E. H. & Chang, J. K. (2000). Orexins: a role in medullary sympathetic outflow. *Regul. Pept.*, *96*, 65-70.

Dutschmann, M., Kron, M., Mörschel, M. & Gestreau, C. (2007). Activation of Orexin B receptors in the pontine Kölliker-Fuse nucleus modulates pre-inspiratory hypoglossal motor activity in rat. *Respir. Physiol. Neurobiol.*, *159*, 232-235.

Elias, C. F., Saper, C. B., Maratos-Flier, E., Tritos, N. A., Lee, C., Kelly, J., Tatro, J. B., Hoffman, G. E., Ollmann, M. M., Barsh, G. S., Sakurai, T., Yanagisawa, M. & Elmquist, J. K. (1998). Chemically defined projections linking the mediobasal hypothalamus and the lateral hypothalamic area. *J. Comp. Neurol.*, *402*, 442-459.

Espana, R. A., Valentino, R. J. & Berridge, C. W. (2003). Fos immunoreactivity in hypocretin-synthesizing and hypocretin-1 receptor-expressing neurons: effects of diurnal and nocturnal spontaneous waking, stress and hypocretin-1 administration. *Neuroscience*, *121*, 201-217.

Feldman, J. L., Mitchell, G. S. & Nattie, E. E. (2003). Breathing: rhythmicity, plasticity, chemosensitivity. *Annu. Rev. Neurosci.*, *26*, 239-266.

Fronczek, R., Overeem, S., Reijntjes, R., Lammers, G., van Dijk, J. & Pijl, H. (2008). Increased heart rate variability but normal resting metabolic rate in hypocretin/orexin-deficient human narcolepsy. *J. Clin. Sleep Med.*, *4*, 248-254.

Fung, S. J., Yamuy, J., Sampogna, S., Morales, F. R. & Chase, M. H. (2001). Hypocretin (orexin) input to trigeminal and hypoglossal motoneurons in the cat: a double-labeling immunohistochemical study. *Brain Res.*, *903*, 257-262.

Geerling, J. C., Mettenleiter, T. C. & Loewy, A. D. (2003). Orexin neurons project to diverse sympathetic outflow systems. *Neuroscience*, *122*, 541-550.

Guilleminault, C. (1993). Amphetamines and narcolepsy: Use of the Stanford database. *Sleep*, *16*, 199-201.

Hakansson, M., de Lecea, L., Sutcliffe, J. G., Yanagisawa, M. & Meister, B. (1999). Leptin receptor- and STAT3-immunoreactivities in hypocretin/ orexin neurones of the lateral hypothalamus. *J. Neuroendocrinol.*, *11*, 653-663.

Hara, J., Beuckmann, C. T., Nambu, T., Willie, J. T., Chemelli, R. M., Sinton, C. M., Sugiyama, F., Yagami, K., Goto, K., Yanagisawa, M. & Sakurai, T. (2001). Genetic ablation of orexin neurons in mice results in narcolepsy, hypophagia, and obesity. *Neuron*, *30*, 345-354.

Harris, G. C. & Aston-Jones, G. (2006). Arousal and reward: a dichotomy in orexin function. *Trends Neurosci.*, *29*, 571-577.

Hess, W. R. (1954). *The Diencephalon: Autonomic and Extrapyramidal Functions.* New York, Grune & Stratton.

Ida, T., Nakahara, K., Murakami, T., Hanada, R., Nakazato, M. & Murakami, N. (2000). Possible involvement of orexin in the stress reaction in rats. *Biochem. Biophys. Res. Commun.*, *270*, 318-323.

Igarashi, N., Tatsumi, K., Nakamura, A., Sakao, S., Takiguchi, Y., Nishikawa, T. & Kuriyama, T. (2003). Plasma orexin-A levels in obstructive sleep apnea-hypopnea syndrome. *Chest*, *124*, 1381-1385.

Jászberényi, M., Bujdosó, E., Pataki, I. & Telegdy, G. (2000). Effects of orexins on the hypothalamic-pituitary-adrenal system. *J. Neuroendocrinol.*, *12*, 1174-1178.

Jordan, A. S. & White, D. P. (2008). Pharyngeal motor control and the pathogenesis of obstructive sleep apnea. *Respir. Physiol. Neurobiol.*, *160*, 1-7.

Jordan, D. (1990). Autonomic changes in affective behavior. In: A. D. Loewy, & K. M. Spyer (Eds.), *Central Regulation of Autonomic Functions*. New York: Oxford University Press, 349-366.

Kanbayashi, T., Inoue, Y., Kawanishi, K., Takasaki, H., Aizawa, R., Takahashi, K., Ogawa, Y., Abe, M., Hishikawa, Y. & Shimizu, T. (2003). CSF hypocretin measures in patients with obstructive sleep apnea. *J. Sleep Res.*, *12*, 339-341.

Kayaba, Y., Nakamura, A., Kasuya, Y., Ohuchi, T., Yanagisawa, M., Komuro, I., Fukuda, Y. & Kuwaki, T. (2003). Attenuated defense response and low basal blood pressure in orexin knockout mice. *Am. J. Physiol. Regul. Integr. Comp. Physiol.*, *285*, R581-R593.

Kiely, J. M. & Gordon, F. J. (1994). Role of rostral ventrolateral medulla in centrally mediated pressor responses *Am. J. Physiol.*, *267*, H1549-H1556.

Krieger, J. (2000). Respiratory physiology: Breathing in normal subjects. In: M. H. Kryger, T. Roth, & W. C. Dement (Eds.), *Principles and Practice of Sleep Medicine*. Philadelphia: W.B. Saunders, 229-241.

Krout, K. E., Mettenleiter, T. C. & Loewy, A. D. (2003). Single CNS neurons link both central motor and cardiosympathetic systems: a double-virus tracing study. *Neuroscience*, *118*, 853-866.

Krout, K. E., Mettenleiter, T. C., Karpitskiy, V., Nguyen, X. V. & Loewy, A. D. (2005). CNS neurons with links to both mood-related cortex and sympathetic nervous system. *Brain Res.*, *1050*, 199-202.

Kumada, M., Terui, N. & Kuwaki, T. (1990). Arterial baroreceptor reflex : its central and peripheral neural mechanisms. *Prog. Neurobiol.*, *35*, 331-361.

Kuwaki, T. (2008). Orexinergic modulation of breathing across vigilance states. *Respir. Physiol. Neurobiol.*, *164*, 204-212.

Kuwaki, T., Deng, B. S., Nakamura, A., Zhang, W., Yanagisawa, M. & Fukuda, Y. (2005). Abnormal respiration in orexin knockout mice. In: A. Kumar, & H. Mallick (Eds.), *Proceedings of the 2nd Interim Congress of the World Federation of Sleep Research and Sleep Medicine Society*. Bologna Italy: Medimond S.r.l., 69-72.

Kuwaki, T., Zhang, W. & Nakamura, A. (2007). State-dependent adjustment of the central autonomic regulation: Role of orexin in emotional behavior and sleep/wake cycle. In: T. Kubo, & T. Kuwaki (Eds.), *Central Mechanisms of Cardiovascular Regulation*. Kerala (India): Research Signport, 57-73.

Kuwaki, T., Zhang, W., Nakamura, A. & Deng, B. (2008). Emotional and state-dependent modification of cardiorespiratory function: role of orexinergic neurons. *Autonom. Neurosci.: Basic Clin.*, *142*, 11-16.

Lee, M., Hassani, O. & Jones, B. (2005). Discharge of identified orexin/hypocretin neurons across the sleep-waking cycle. *J. Neurosci.*, *25*, 6716-6720.

Machado, B. H., Bonagamba, L. G., Dun, S. L., Kwok, E. H. & Dun, N. J. (2002). Pressor response to microinjection of orexin/hypocretin into rostral ventrolateral medulla of awake rats. *Regul. Pept.*, *104*, 75-81.

Mileykovskiy, B., Kiyashchenko, L. & Siegel, J. (2005). Behavioral correlates of activity in identified hypocretin/orexin neurons. *Neuron*, *46*, 787-798.

Millhorn, D. E., Eldridge, F. L. & Waldrop, T. G. (1980). Prolonged stimulation of respiration by a new central neural mechanism. *Respir. Physiol.*, *41*, 87-103.

Mitchell, G. S. & Johnson, S. M. (2003). Neuroplasticity in respiratory motor control. *J. Appl. Physiol.*, *94*, 358-374.

Nakamura, A. & Kuwaki, T. (2004). Sleep apnea in mice: A useful animal model for study of SIDS? *Pathophysiology*, *10*, 253-257.

Nakamura, A., Fukuda, Y. & Kuwaki, T. (2003). Sleep apnea and effect of chemostimulation on breathing instability in mice. *J. Appl. Physiol.*, *94*, 525-532.

Nakamura, A., Zhang, W., Yanagisawa, M., Fukuda, Y. & Kuwaki, T. (2007). Vigilance state-dependent attenuation of hypercapnic chemoreflex and exaggerated sleep apnea in orexin knockout mice. *J. Appl. Physiol.*, *102*, 241-248.

Nalivaiko, E., Ootsuka, Y. & Blessing, W. W. (2005). Activation of 5-HT1A receptors in the medullary raphe reduces cardiovascular changes elicited by acute psychological and inflammatory stresses in rabbits. *Am. J. Physiol. Regul. Integr. Comp. Physiol.*, *289*, R596-R604.

Nambu, T., Sakurai, T., Mizukami, K., Hosoya, Y., Yanagisawa, M. & Goto, K. (1999). Distribution of orexin neurons in the adult rat brain. *Brain Res.*, *827*, 243-260.

Nosaka, S. (1996). Modifications of arterial baroreflexes: obligatory roles in cardiovascular regulation in stress and poststress recovery. *Jpn. J. Physiol.*, *46*, 271-288.

Peyron, C., Tighe, D. K., van den Pol, A. N., de Lecea, L., Heller, H. C., Sutcliffe, J. G. & Kilduff, T. S. (1998). Neurons containing hypocretin (orexin) project to multiple neuronal systems. *J. Neurosci.*, *18*, 9996-10015.

Phillipson, E. (1978). Control of breathing during sleep. *Am. Rev. Respir. Dis.*, *118*, 909-939.

Pitkanen, A., Savander, V. & LeDoux, J. E. (1997). Organization of intra-amygdaloid circuitries in the rat: an emerging framework for understanding functions of the amygdala. *Trends Neurosci.*, *20*, 517-523.

Polotsky, V. Y., Wilson, J. A., Haines, A. S., Scharf, M. T., Soutiere, S. E., Tankersley, C. G., Smith, P. L., Schwartz, A. R. & O'Donnell, C. P. (2001). The impact of insulin-dependent diabetes on ventilatory control in the mouse. *Am. J. Respir. Crit. Care Med.*, *163*, 624-632.

Powell, F. L., Milsom, W. K. & Mitchell, G. S. (1998). Time domains of the hypoxic ventilatory response. *Respir. Physiol.*, *112*, 123-134.

Punjabi, N. M., Shahar, E., Rediline, S., Gottlieb, D. J., Givelber, R., Resnick, H. E. & Sleep Heat Health Study Investigators. (2004). Sleep-disordered breathing, glucose intolerance, and insulin resistance: the Sleep Heart Health Study. *Am. J. Epidemiol.*, *160*, 521-530.

Rosin, D. L., Chang, D. A. & Guyenet, P. G. (2006). Afferent and efferent connections of the rat retrotrapezoid nucleus. *J. Comp. Neurol.*, *499*, 64-89.

Rosin, D. L., Weston, M. C., Sevigny, C. P., Stornetta, R. L. & Guyenet, P. G. (2003). Hypothalamic orexin (hypocretin) neurons express vesicular glutamate transporters VGLUT1 or VGLUT2. *J. Comp. Neurol.*, *465*, 593-603.

Sachs, C. & Kaijser, L. (1982). Autonomic regulation of cardiopulmonary functions in sleep apnea syndrome and narcolepsy. *Sleep*, *5*, 227-238.

Sakurai, S., Nishijima, T., Takahashi, S., Yamauchi, K., Arihara, Z. & Takahashi, K. (2005a). Low plasma orexin-A levels were improved by continuous positive airway pressure treatment in patients with severe obstructive sleep apnea-hypopnea syndrome. *Chest*, *127*, 731-737.

Sakurai, T. (2007). The neural circuit of orexin (hypocretin): maintaining sleep and wakefulness. *Nat. Rev. Neurosci.*, *8*, 171-181.

Sakurai, T., Amemiya, A., Ishii, M., Matsuzaki, I., Chemelli, R. M., Tanaka, H., Williams, S. C., Richarson, J. A., Kozlowski, G. P., Wilson, S., Arch, J. R., Buckingham, R. E., Haynes, A. C., Carr, S. A., Annan, R. S., McNulty, D. E., Liu, W. S., Terrett, J. A., Elshourbagy, N. A., Bergsma, D. J. & Yanagisawa, M. (1998). Orexins and orexin receptors: a family of hypothalamic neuropeptides and G protein-coupled receptors that regulate feeding behavior. *Cell*, *92*, 573-585.

Sakurai, T., Nagata, R., Yamanaka, A., Kawamura, H., Tsujino, N., Muraki, Y., Kageyama, H., Kunita, S., Takahashi, S., Goto, K., Koyama, Y., Shioda, S. &

Yanagisawa, M. (2005b). Input of orexin/hypocretin neurons revealed by a genetically encoded tracer in mice. *Neuron*, *46*, 297-308.

Samson, W. K., Gosnell, B., Chang, J. K., Resch, Z. T. & Murphy, T. C. (1999). Cardiovascular regulatory actions of the hypocretins in brain. *Brain Res.*, *831*, 248-253.

Saper, C. B., Scammell, T. E. & Lu, J. (2005). Hypothalamic regulation of sleep and circadian rhythms. *Nature*, *437*, 1257-1263.

Sévoz-Couche, C., Comet, M. A., Hamon, M. & Laguzzi, R. (2003). Role of nucleus tractus solitarius 5-HT3 receptors in the defense reaction-induced inhibition of the aortic baroreflex in rats. . *J. Neurophysiol.*, *90*, 2521-2530.

Shirasaka, T., Nakazato, M., Matsukura, S., Takasaki, M. & Kannan, H. (1999). Sympathetic and cardiovascular actions of orexins in conscious rats. *Am. J. Physiol.*, *277*, R1780-R1785.

Smart, D., Sabido-David, C., Brough, S. J., Jewitt, F., Johns, A., Porter, R. A. & Jerman, J. C. (2001). SB-334867-A: the first selective orexin-1 receptor antagonist. *Br. J. Pharmacol.*, *132*, 1179-1182.

Smith, B. N., Davis, S. F., Van Den Pol, A. N. & Xu, W. (2002). Selective enhancement of excitatory synaptic activity in the rat nucleus tractus solitarius by hypocretin 2. *Neuroscience*, *115*, 707-714.

Sun, M. K. & Guyenet, P. G. (1986). Hypothalamic glutamatergic input to medullary sympathoexcitatory neurons in rats. *Am. J. Physiol.*, *251*, R798-R810.

Sunanaga, J., Deng, B., Zhang, W., Kanmura, Y. & Kuwaki, T. (2009). CO2 activates orexin-containing neurons in mice. *Respir. Physiol. Neurobiol.*, *166*, 184-186.

Terada, J., Nakamura, A., Zhang, W., Yanagisawa, M., Kuriyama, T., Fukuda, Y. & Kuwaki, T. (2008). Ventilatory long-term facilitation in mice can be observed both during sleep and wake periods and depends on orexin. *J. Appl. Physiol.*, *104*, 499-507.

Thannickal, T. C., Moore, R. Y., Nienhuis, R., Ramanathan, L., Gulyani, S., Aldrich, M., Cornford, M. & Siegel, J. M. (2000). Reduced number of hypocretin neurons in human narcolepsy. *Neuron*, *27*, 469-474.

Thomas, T. & Spyer, K. M. (1996). The role of adenosine receptors in the rostral ventrolateral medulla in the cardiovascular response to defence area stimulation in the rat. *Exp. Physiol.*, *81*, 67-77.

Volgin, D. V., Saghir, M. & Kubin, L. (2002). Developmental changes in the orexin 2 receptor mRNA in hypoglossal motoneurons. *Neuroreport*, *13*, 433-436.

Watanabe, S., Kuwaki, T., Yanagisawa, M., Fukuda, Y. & Shimoyama, M. (2005). Persistent pain and stress activate pain-inhibitory orexin pathways. *Neuroreport*, *16*, 5-8.

Williams, R. H., Jensen, L. T., Verkhratsky, A., Fugger, L. & Burdakov, D. (2007). Control of hypothalamic orexin neurons by acid and CO2. *Proc. Natl. Acad. Sci.*, USA., *104*, 10685-10690.

Willie, J. T., Chemelli, R. M., Sinton, C. M. & Yanagisawa, M. (2001). To eat or to sleep? Orexin in the regulation of feeding and wakefulness. *Annu. Rev. Neurosci.*, *24*, 429-458.

Winsky-Sommerer, R., Yamanaka, A., Diano, S., Borok, E., Roberts, A. J., Sakurai, T., Kilduff, T. S., Horvath, T. L. & de Lecea, L. (2004). Interaction between the corticotropin-releasing factor system and hypocretins (orexins): a novel circuit mediating stress response. *J. Neurosci.*, *24*, 11439-11448.

Yamamoto, T., Nozaki-Taguchi, N. & Chiba, T. (2002). Analgesic effect of intrathecally administered orexin-A in the rat formalin test and in the rat hot plate test. *Br. J. Pharmacol.*, *137*, 170-176.

Yamanaka, A., Beuckmann, C. T., Willie, J. T., Hara, J., Tsujino, N., Mieda, M., Tominaga, M., Yagami, K., Sugiyama, F., Goto, K., Yanagisawa, M. & Sakurai, T. (2003). Hypothalamic orexin neurons regulate arousal according to energy balance in mice. *Neuron*, *38*, 701-713.

Yoshida, K., McCormack, S., Espana, R. A., Crocker, A. & Scammell, T. E. (2006). Afferents to the orexin neurons of the rat brain. *J. Comp. Neurol.*, *494*, 845-861.

Young, J. K., Wu, M., Manaye, K. F., Kc, P., Allard, J. S., Mack, S. O. & Haxhiu, M. A. (2005). Orexin stimulates breathing via medullary and spinal pathways. *J. Appl. Physiol.*, *98*, 1387-1395.

Zhang, W., Fukuda, Y. & Kuwaki, T. (2005). Respiratory and cardiovascular actions of orexin-A in mice. *Neurosci. Lett.*, *385*, 131-136.

Zhang, W., Sakurai, T., Fukuda, Y. & Kuwaki, T. (2006a). Orexin neuron-mediated skeletal muscle vasodilation and shift of baroreflex during defense response in mice. *Am. J. Physiol. Regul. Integr. Comp. Physiol.*, *290*, R1654-R1663.

Zhang, W., Shimoyama, M., Fukuda, Y. & Kuwaki, T. (2006b). Multiple components of the defense response depend on orexin: Evidence from orexin knockout mice and orexin neuron-ablated mice. *Autonom. Neurosci.: Basic Clin.*, *126-127*, 139-145.

Zhang, W., Zhang, N., Sakurai, T. & Kuwaki, T. (2009). Orexin neurons in the hypothalamus mediate cardiorespiratory responses induced by disinhibition of thc amygdala and bed nucleus of the stria terminalis. *Brain Res.*, *1262*, 25-37.

Zhu, L., Onaka, T., Sakurai, T. & Yada, T. (2002). Activation of orexin neurones after noxious but not conditioned fear stimuli in rats. *Neuroreport*, *13*, 1351-1353.

In: Nacrolepsy: Symptoms, Causes...
Editors: G. Santos et al. pp. 35-64
ISBN: 978-1-60876-645-1

Chapter II

Modafinil: A Wake-Promoting Stimulant with Multiple Clinical Uses

***Dennis K. Miller*[1*] *and Marsha M. Dopheide*[2]**
[1]Department of Psychological Sciences and Bond Life Sciences Center, University of Missouri, Columbia MO.
[2]Department of Psychology, Monmouth College, Monmouth IL.

Abstract

Modafinil is a mild, wake-promoting stimulant that is pharmacologically distinct from other central nervous system stimulants. Modafinil is approved in the United States for the treatment of narcolepsy and has been demonstrated to be effective and well-tolerated. Modafinil also has been approved for use in treating shift work sleep disorder and as an adjunctive treatment for obstructive sleep apnea/hypopnea syndrome. Similar to other stimulants, modafinil increases arousal and has cognitive benefits. Beyond managing sleep disorders, modafinil has been used to manage the symptoms of Attention-Deficit Hyperactivity Disorder, depression, schizophrenia, and addiction to cocaine and amphetamines. The findings with human subjects

* Corresponding author: Department of Psychological Sciences, McAlester Hall, University of Missouri, Columbia MO 65211, Email: millerden@missouri.edu, Telephone: 573-884-8141, Fax: 573-882-7710.

have been supported by basic animal behavioral research. Despite modafinil's numerous clinical uses, its mechanism of action in the brain is unclear: Modafinil interacts with multiple targets in the central nervous system—dopamine, norepinephrine, serotonin and orexin receptors—associated with modafinil's clinical and behavioral effects. The present chapter offers an overview of modafinil's effects on human and animal behavior and in the brain.

Introduction

Psychomotor stimulants are used for a variety of therapeutic purposes, such as for the treatment of narcolepsy and attention deficit hyperactivity disorder (ADHD) and to sustain general arousal. Examples of therapeutic stimulants in the United States (US) include the amphetamines (*d*-, *l*- and *dl*-amphetamine; trade names include Benzedrine, Dexedrine and Adderall), methylphenidate (Ritalin), cocaine (used therapeutically as an anesthetic), methamphetamine (used infrequently for ADHD as Desoxyn) and modafinil (2-[di(phenyl)methylsulfinyl]acetamide; Provigil, Alertec, and Vigiler). Stimulants can have a number of side effects—such as psychosis, motor agitation and restlessness, and abuse and dependence—that have limited their use. Within the body, stimulants increase monoamine (dopamine, norepinephrine and serotonin) synaptic transmission and activate the sympathetic nervous system or mimic sympathetic arousal.

In the US modafinil is approved by the Food and Drug Administration (see www.fda.gov) to manage the symptoms of sleep disorders, such as narcolepsy, obstructive sleep apnea syndrome and shift-work sleep disorder (SWSD) (for review see Ballon & Feifel, 2006; Kumar, 2008). There are a number of off-label and/or experimental uses for modafinil including, but not limited to, ADHD, depression, schizophrenia and cocaine and amphetamine dependence. Modafinil has been marketed in the US for over a decade (since 1998) for these purposes and has generally been effective with relatively-few side effects that would limit its use (Spiller et al., 2009). An active enantiomer (Armodafinil, (-)-2-[(R)-(diphenylmethyl)sulfinyl]acetamide) of the racemic modafinil has recently been introduced in the US and has pharmacological properties similar to modafinil (Lankford, 2008).

Pharmacologically, modafinil is considered to be a "mild" stimulant because it is less potent and efficacious than other stimulants (e.g., amphetamine, methamphetamine and cocaine) (Dopheide, Morgan, Rodvelt, Schachtman, & Miller, 2007; Zolkowska et al., 2009). While considered relatively mild and safe, modafinil is a prescription drug in the US and is a Schedule IV controlled substance under the US Comprehensive Drug Abuse Prevention and Control Act (see www.usdoj.gov/dea). This classification designates modafinil as a drug with an accepted medical use, low potential for abuse, but it may have limited potential for physical or psychological dependence. For comparison, the stronger stimulants (e.g., amphetamine, cocaine and methlylphenidate) are classified as Schedule II substances, indicating an accepted medical use, but high abuse potential and possibility for dependence. Throughout this chapter, modafinil will be compared to the other, "stronger" stimulants.

A review of the US National Library of Medicine's PubMed database (www.pubmed.gov) of the scientific and medical literature in summer 2009 revealed over 750 citations for research and clinical articles on modafinil. This chapter does not comment on each of these reports, but rather it summarizes the basic research on modafinil, with a focus on its indication to minimize the daytime sleepiness and drowsiness associated with sleep disorders. Comments on its off-label uses (e.g., ADHD and mood disorders) and potential side effects (e.g., drug abuse and dependence) also are presented here to present an overview of this drug with a very interesting pharmacological profile.

Modafinil in Sleep Disorders

The American Psychiatric Association's Diagnostic and Statistical Manual of Mental Disorders (DSM-IV; see www.psychiatryonline.com) recognizes a number sleep disorders. These can be characterized as abnormalities in the amount, quality or timing of sleep (collectively labeled dyssomnias), and abnormalities in sleep behavior or events that occur during sleep (parasomnias). Modafinil is indicated for the management of the symptoms of and/or outcomes from dyssomnias such as narcolepsy, obstructive sleep apnea syndrome (a Breathing-Related Sleep Disorder in the DSM-IV) and SWSD (known as Circadian Rhythm Sleep Disorder in the DSM-IV).

Narcolepsy

Narcolepsy is a sleep disorder characterized by excessive daytime sleepiness that is present even if the individual experiences a restful night's sleep. The individual experiences extreme fatigue, drowsiness, and a strong urge to nap at inappropriate times throughout the day. Cataplexy, sleep paralysis and hypnagogic hallucinations may also be present. The symptoms of narcolepsy are related to diminished orexin release in the hypothalamus, and can be managed with stimulants such as amphetamine, methylphenidate or modafinil.

Numerous studies have demonstrated modafinil's effectiveness in treating the excessive daytime sleepiness associated with narcolepsy (Ballon & Feifel, 2006; Schwartz, 2005). The US Modafinil in Narcolepsy Study Group (1998; 2000), in double-blind, placebo-controlled studies, found that modafinil (200-400 mg, peroral [p.o.] administration) improved scores on three different measures of sleep and prolonged wakefulness. These findings are supported by other trials, where subjects given modafinil (200, 300, or 400 mg, p.o.) generally experienced significant reductions in daytime sleepiness and daytime sleep, with few changes in nighttime sleepiness or other significant effects (Billiard et al., 1994; Broughton et al., 1997; Schwartz, Feldman, & Bogan, 2005).

The modafinil doses employed in these studies (200-400 mg, p.o.) appear high, relative to other stimulants used to manage sleep disorders (e.g., ~20-50 mg p.o. for *d*-amphetamines). However, adverse effects and side effects are relatively uncommon within this dose range (Spiller et al., 2009). Typical side effects include agitation, irritability and anxiety. Physiological side effects of headache, gastrointestinal distress and skin irritation also have been reported, although these generally diminish with reduction of the dose or splitting the dosage to twice-a-day administration. Physical or physiological withdrawal symptoms have not been reported with modafinil (Ballon & Feifel, 2006; Spiller et al., 2009). While modafinil is a stimulant, it lacks some of the reinforcing properties observed with more-potent stimulants (e.g., amphetamines) (Rush, Kelly, Hays, & Wooten, 2002; Rush, Kelly, Hays, Baker, & Wooten, 2002), which minimizes, but doesn't eliminate, its abuse and dependence potential

Taken together, research investigating modafinil's effectiveness in individuals with narcolepsy demonstrate that it is an effective and well-tolerated wake-promoting agent. While modafinil is effective to reduce sleepiness during the day, it has not shown usefulness in treating other symptoms of narcolepsy--cataplexy, sleep paralysis and hypnogogic hallucinations. Other medications (e.g., antidepressants, antipsychotics or sedatives) would be more effective for managing these other symptoms (Billiard, 2008).

Obstructive Sleep Apnea Syndrome

Obstructive sleep apnea is characterized by frequent blockages of the upper airway during sleep. These blockages disrupt night time sleep, which may lead to excessive daytime sleepiness. While other stimulants (e.g., amphetamines and ephedrine) act as vasodilators and bronchodilators, modafinil has not been shown to overcome airway blockage. However, it (200 and 400 mg, p.o.) has minimized the daytime sleepiness in sleep apnea (Bittencourt et al., 2008; Black & Hirshkowitz, 2005; Pack, Black, Schwartz, & Matheson, 2001). In addition, modafinil can restore performance on cognitive and behavioral tasks impaired by daytime sleepiness (Bittencourt et al., 2008). In contrast to the positive findings with modafinil, Kingshott and colleagues (2001) found no significant difference between individuals given modafinil (400 mg, p.o.) and those given placebo on restoration of cognitive functions impaired following sleep apnea, even though modafinil decreased daytime sleepiness. In summary, modafinil may be an effective treatment for the daytime sleepiness that occurs in individuals with sleep apnea; however, any potential cognitive benefits need to be further explored.

Shift-work Sleep Disorder (Circadian Rhythm Sleep Disorder)

SWSD is a circadian rhythm disturbance that often affects individuals with an inconsistent daily work schedule or who work overnight more than during the day. Typically, individuals with SWSD suffer from insomnia or excessive sleepiness, the latter of which responds well to treatment with modafinil (Ballon & Feifel, 2006). In a double-blind, placebo-controlled study (Czeisler et al., 2005), modafinil (200 mg, p.o.) improved vigilance, as well as reduced subjective ratings of sleepiness. Despite these benefits; however, subjects showed no differences in sleep episodes, accidents, or caffeine consumption at work. In a separate study (Walsh, Randazzo, Stone, & Schweitzer, 2004), individuals with SWSD were administered modafinil (200 mg, p.o.) or placebo for four consecutive nights followed by 6-8 hours of daytime sleep. Compared to placebo, modafinil improved performance on some cognitive tasks normally impaired by sleepiness. At this point, it is still unclear whether modafinil is globally beneficial to individuals suffering from SWSD or if its usefulness is limited to treating only certain symptoms of the disorder, such as improving wakefulness and attention.

Wake-promoting and Cognitive-enhancing Effects

Beyond its use in individuals with narcolepsy, sleep apnea or SWSD, modafinil's wake-promoting effects for other dyssomnias are documented. For example, in healthy subjects, modafinil (300 mg, p.o.) increased alertness similar to amphetamine (20 mg, p.o.) (Chapotot, Pigeau, Canini, Bourdon, & Buguet, 2003). One study (Wesensten, Killgore, & Balkin, 2005) evaluated the relative efficacy of caffeine (600 mg, p.o.), amphetamine (20 mg, p.o.), and modafinil (400 mg, p.o.) for restoring and maintaining cognitive performance in healthy young adults after three nights of sleep deprivation. All three drugs were comparable for improving response speed on a vigilance task up to 6 hours post-administration and for maintaining wakefulness up to 2 hours after administration. All three drugs also improved some aspects of executive function.

Modafinil has been used by soldiers during prolonged military operations when natural circadian rhythms may be affected or when pilots are kept awake over long hours and unable to fulfill their need for sleep (Eliyahu, Berlin, Hadad, Heled, & Moran, 2007). Using a demanding flight-stimulator to explore the cognitive-enhancing effects of modafinil in normal, sleep-deprived volunteers, modafinil (200 mg, p.o.) was shown to be effective in sustaining performance and alertness when compared to placebo (Caldwell, Jr., Caldwell, Smythe, III, & Hall, 2000). Historically, amphetamines have been used for these military and aviation purposes, but Eliyahu and colleagues (2007) reported that modafinil has efficacy similar to amphetamines, and with fewer side effects. A combination of modafinil with short naps over prolonged operations may have greater success to counter fatigue than wither approach, modafinil or naps, alone (Batejat & Lagarde, 1999; Caldwell, Jr. et al., 2000).

In the absence of sleep deprivation or disruption of circadian rhythms, the ability of modafinil to improve cognition is much more ambiguous than its known ability to enhance wakefulness (Minzenberg & Carter, 2008). Some studies have found evidence of enhanced cognitive performance--working memory, impulse control, vigilance and sustained attention--in healthy volunteers (e.g., individuals without a sleep disorder). For example, Turner and colleagues (2003) showed that modafinil (200 mg, p.o.) enhanced performance on tests of digital span, visual pattern recognition memory, spatial planning and stop-signal reaction time in young males. While enhancing performance, modafinil also slowed reaction time (i.e., increased response latencies), a seemingly speed-accuracy trade off. Thus, modafinil appears to enhance accuracy, perhaps inhibiting impulsive responding as evidenced by slower reaction times. Others have found little evidence of any modafinil-induced cognitive improvement in non sleep-deprived individuals. Liepert and colleagues (2004) did not find any effect of modafinil (200 mg, p.o.) on dexterity, attention and concentration, or motor excitability in healthy adults. Randall and colleagues (2003) also failed to detect any positive findings of modafinil (100 and 200 mg, p.o.) on cognitive performance in healthy adults. Furthermore, tests of reaction time and tasks that focused on attention control were not affected by modafinil at all (Muller, Steffenhagen, Regenthal, & Bublak, 2004). Thus, positive effects of modafinil on cognitive performance have not consistently been found in the absence of sleep problems.

To date, it remains unclear whether these discrepant findings are due to a lack of drug efficacy in healthy adults, small sample sizes in various studies, or from differences in task difficulty or sensitivity in these studies. Further research is required to make any definitive conclusions about modafinil as a true general cognition enhancer. At present, it seems that modafinil does not act as an enhancer; but it may selectively improve task performance, especially if performance is compromised by sleep deprivation or by some pathology. This is an important question considering anecdotal reports of modafinil to help college students study and prepare for exams (see www.provigilweb.org/ upallnight.htm).

Summary

Modafinil is effective to manage the symptoms of and/or outcomes from dyssomnias. It minimizes the excessive daytime sleepiness observed in narcolepsy, sleep apnea and in SWSD. It also can reverse some of the cognitive deficits associated with fatigue, sleepiness and an irregular circadian rhythm.

Modafinil on Other Psychiatric Disorders

Modafinil also has a number of off-label uses and is being investigated to manage the symptoms of several psychological disorders (Teitelman, 2001). This section briefly comments on modafinil's use in ADHD, depression, bipolar disorder and schizophrenia, and drug addiction. Other off-label or experimental uses for modafinil include alleviating the muscle fatigue in multiple sclerosis, improving athletic performance, and aiding weight loss for the obese (Kumar, 2008).

Attention Deficit Hyperactivity Disorder

ADHD is a persistent pattern of inattention or hyperactivity that is more intense than typically observed at that developmental level. The symptoms of ADHD are typically treated with amphetamines (Adderall) and methylphenidate (Concerta or Ritalin). These stronger stimulants minimize ADHD's symptoms by increasing alertness (Gonon, 2009); however, the pharmacological strength of amphetamines and methylphenidate may contribute to undesired side effects that are absent with the milder stimulant modafinil. Several clinical studies have investigated modafinil to manage the symptoms of ADHD (Lindsay, Gudelsky, & Heaton, 2006; Minzenberg & Carter, 2008). In one double-blind placebo-controlled study, amphetamine and modafinil (~209 mg, p.o.) were equally effective in managing the symptoms of ADHD in adults (Taylor & Russo, 2000). Furthermore, two separate studies indicated that modafinil (~170-425 mg/kg, PO) improved children's ratings on measures of sustained attention and other behavioral rating scales (Rugino & Copley, 2001; Rugino & Samsock, 2003). Based on these and other findings, the drug company Cephalon sought approval from the US Food and Drug Administration in the mid-2000s to market modafinil as a treatment for the symptoms of ADHD in children. However, approval was not given to Cephalon, due to concerns over potential side effects.

Depression

In addition to low mood, anhedonia and thoughts of death, the symptoms of depression can include sleep and arousal disturbances (e.g., hypersomnia, insomnia and/or feelings of fatigue). Modafinil has been shown to be effective to manage these sleep-related symptoms (Lam, Freeman, & Cates, 2007; Orr & Taylor, 2007). When added as an adjunct to typical antidepressant therapy, modafinil (200 mg/day, p.o.) improved depression-associated lethargy and somnolence in patients who were only partially responsive to their original treatment of antidepressants alone (Markovitz & Wagner, 2003). Aside from a reduction in fatigue, patients have also expressed an improvement in cognitive and physical functioning (Fava, Thase, & DeBattista, 2005; Menza, Kaufman, & Castellanos, 2000).

Few studies have addressed modafinil's usefulness as a monotherapy in treating depression. In one case report (Kaufman, Menza, & Fitzsimmons, 2002), a patient did not respond well to treatments with three typically-used antidepressants because of either minimal medication response or intolerable side effects. Many depression symptoms (e.g., decreased energy, interest, concentration, and memory) were reported to be less severe after one week of modafinil (200 mg, p.o.) treatment.

Bipolar Disorder and Schizophrenia

Bipolar disorder is characterized by intermittent periods of mania and schizophrenia consists of abnormalities in the perception of reality. Stimulants are traditionally associated with the risk of worsening or precipitating disorder symptoms. For example, one report implicated modafinil as the trigger for a first manic episode in a boy being treated for narcolepsy (Vorspan, Warot, Consoli, Cohen, & Mazet, 2005). However, modafinil produced a facilitative effect on cognition in individuals with schizophrenia. Studies conducted by Rosenthal and Bryant (2004) and Turner and colleagues (2004) both reported a positive effect on cognition when modafinil (200 mg, p.o.) was added to an antipsychotic regimen. However, others have found that similar doses of modafinil did not result in any change in schizophrenia's symptoms (Sevy et al., 2005).

Stimulant Abuse and Dependence

Considering that modafinil increases wakefulness and arousal and might be reinforcing or rewarding, its abuse (a maladaptive pattern of drug use that leads to problems in day-to-day life in the DSM-IV) and dependence (characterized by tolerance and withdrawal in the DSM-IV) liability is a matter of great concern. In assessing a drug's abuse potential, researchers investigate the degree to which that compound shares characteristics with known addictive drugs (e.g., amphetamines or cocaine). Modafinil's (300 mg, p.o.) subjective effects were compared with those of amphetamine (15 mg, p.o.), caffeine (300 mg, p.o.) and placebo in healthy adults with no history of drug abuse or dependence, and moderate use of caffeine (Warot, Corruble, Payan, Weil, & Puech, 1993). Subjects reported modafinil and caffeine, but not modafinil and amphetamine, to be subjectively similar. Only amphetamine increased feelings of euphoria and a sense of well-being often associated with abuse. In two separate studies (Rush et al., 2002; Rush et al., 2002), modafinil failed to produce effects indicative of abuse potential in individuals with a recent history of cocaine use. For example, in one study, subjects were trained to discriminate cocaine (250 mg, p.o.) from placebo, and then administered cocaine (50, 100, or 150 mg, p.o.), modafinil (200, 400, 600 mg, p.o.) or placebo. Modafinil did not produce cocaine-like discriminative responses.

In contrast to the above findings, Stoops and colleagues (2005) used a modified progressive ratio procedure and found that the reinforcing effects of modafinil were dose-dependently (0, 100, 200, and 400 mg, p.o.) influenced by the behavioral demands following drug administration. Modafinil was reinforcing under a "performance" condition in which subjects were asked to complete arithmetic problems, but not under a "relaxation" condition, in which subjects were asked to sit quietly, semi-reclined in a darkened room. This suggests that modafinil will function as a reinforcer under taxing or perhaps stressful conditions.

As modafinil shares some of the pharmacological properties (e.g., increased arousal) of addictive stimulants, but lacks these stimulants' abuse and dependence liabilities, modafinil has been investigated as a potential treatment for stimulant abuse and dependence (Sofuoglu & Kosten, 2006; Vocci & Elkashef, 2005).

Dackis and colleagues (2003; 2005) investigated drug interactions between cocaine (30 mg, p.o.) and modafinil (200 and 400 mg, p.o.) in a double-blind placebo-controlled study. When taken with cocaine, modafinil decreased the euphoria associated with cocaine use; however, this effect was significant only for the low (200 mg, p.o.) modafinil dose. Unlike cocaine, modafinil by itself did not increase vital sign responses (i.e., blood pressure, pulse and temperature). Hart and colleagues (2008) recently demonstrated results similar to these earlier findings, as modafinil (200 and 400 mg, p.o.) attenuated smoked cocaine (12-25 mg) self-administration, and positive subjective ratings, and cocaine's cardiovascular effects. This modafinil dose range also has been shown to be effective to increase the number of days between cocaine use and decrease craving for cocaine in patients in a cocaine addiction treatment clinic (Scammell et al., 2000; Anderson et al., 2009).

Regarding other abused stimulants, Shearer and colleagues (2009) reported that modafinil (200 mg, p.o.) did not markedly change methamphetamine craving or the severity of dependence on methamphetamine, but methamphetamine uses administered modafinil were more likely to have methamphetamine-negative urine samples at weekly evaluations than users treated with placebo. Schnoll and colleagues (2008) determined that modafinil was ineffective to decrease tobacco cigarette smoking.

Summary

Modafinil decreases the symptoms of psychiatric disorders, beyond sleep-related disorders. It minimizes ADHD symptoms, although it has not been approved for this purpose in the US. It may also minimize some of the symptoms of depression and schizophrenia. Recently, modafinil has received interest as a treatment for amphetamine and cocaine abuse and dependence. These multiple uses may be related to its multifaceted interaction with man targets in the nervous system (see MODAFINIL'S MECHANISM OF ACTION, below). Finally, while modafinil is a stimulant, it lacks some of the reinforcing properties observed with more-potent stimulants.

Animal Research with Modafinil

Aside from clinical research, many behavioral scientists have investigated modafinil in animals. Animal research has investigated both the behavioral stimulant, cognitive, and potentially-reinforcing effects of modafinil with findings similar to and different from those with human subjects.

Arousal

Stimulants produce a dose- and time-dependent increase in locomotor activity following administration to animals. Modafinil increases locomotor activity following administration to mice (4-256 mg/kg, intraperitoneal [i.p.] or p.o.), rats (20-60 mg/kg, intravenous [i.v.]) and monkeys (16-64 mg/kg, p.o.) (Duteil et al., 1990; Zolkowska et al., 2009). However, modafinil is less potent and efficacious than other stimulants at increasing locomotor activity, and other studies have shown a very modest or no effect of modafinil on activity in animals (Edgar & Seidel, 1997; Simon, Hemet, & Costentin, 1996).

Modafinil has long been known to increase wakefulness in many animals including rodents , cats (Lin et al., 1992), dogs (Shelton, Nishino, Vaught, Dement, & Mignot, 1995), and monkeys (Hermant, Rambert, & Duteil, 1991; Lagarde & Milhaud, 1990). Edgar and Seidel (1997) examined the relationships between drug-induced waking, motor activity as a function of wake time, and subsequent compensatory sleep responses in the rat. Methamphetamine (1 mg/kg, i.p.) and modafinil (300 mg/kg, i.p.) increased total wake time in rats to a similar degree, although modafinil produced longer bouts of continuous wakefulness than methamphetamine. Unlike methamphetamine, modafinil did not elicit strong compensatory sleep responses (i.e., rebound hypersomnolence) after drug-induced waking. Similar patterns of behavior and/or comparisons between modafinil and other stimulants have been reported by Langarde and Milhaud (1990), Hermant and colleagues (1991), Lin and colleagues (1992) and Touret and colleagues (1995).

Animal behavioral research supports clinical research indicating that modafinil is an effective stimulant; yet, it has fewer of the peripheral side effects seen with the more potent stimulants, like amphetamine. Modafinil is effective at increasing arousal, like amphetamine, but it is less potent and efficacious to increase locomotor activity, produce compensatory sleep responses, or increase anxiety (Simon, Panissaud, & Costentin, 1994). This specificity further differentiates modafinil from other stimulants, supporting its viability for individuals sensitive to the side effects of the amphetamine-like drugs.

Learning and Cognition

As indicated, it is controversial whether modafinil improves cognitive performance in non sleep-deprived humans (Turner et al., 2003; Minzenberg & Carter, 2008; Liepert, Allstadt-Schmitz, & Weiller, 2004). Animal researchers have investigated modafinil's effects on cognition and learning, and the role of drug-induced arousal in these processes.

One common test used to assess attention processes in animals is the 5-choice serial reaction time task, which measures various aspects of visual-spatial attention including selective, divided and sustained attention, and response control. Waters and colleagues (2005) observed that modafinil (32-128 mg/kg, i.p.) did not increase impulse control under standard conditions. In fact, in direct contrast to the clinical findings described above, modafinil actually attenuated impulse control under conditions of greater attention load (i.e., increased premature responses). Using middle-aged rats in a similar study, Morgan and colleagues (2007) found results to the contrary. In this study, modafinil (8-64 mg/kg, p.o.) produced a dose-dependent pattern of improved response accuracy, improved impulse control (i.e., decreased premature responses) and shorter response latencies. Furthermore, modafinil did not negatively affect omission errors, motivation or motor control. Importantly, a series of studies by Beracochea and colleagues (2001; 2002; 2003) demonstrated that acute or repeated systemic modafinil (8-64 mg/kg) exposure in healthy adult mice produced enhancement of serial-reversal learning, spatial learning, and working memory that was dependent on task difficulty and baseline stress levels.

Taken together, these studies suggest that modafinil has positive effects on a variety of attention, learning, and memory processes. The magnitude of modaifinil's effects on learning, memory and cognition was dependent, partially, on factors such as age, external stressors and task difficulty. For example, in tasks with little difficulty modafinil impaired performance, but, modafinil enhanced performance in more-difficult tasks. Additional behavior work is required to confirm the observations in humans that modafinil is most effective to reverse or minimize the effects of fatigue on performance.

Drug Addiction

Considering the abuse and dependence liability of stimulants and modafinil's experimental use as a treatment for drug addiction (Sofuoglu & Kosten, 2006; Vocci & Elkashef, 2005), animal research has investigated modafinil's effects in animal models of drug addiction.

In the drug self-administration procedure, in which animals learn to make a response (e.g., press a lever) for i.v. drug infusion, animals learned to respond for cocaine infusion (Deroche-Gamonet et al., 2002; Gold & Balster, 1996). Gold and Balster (1996) observed that modafinil (0.03-0.3 mg/kg, i.v.) was self-administered by monkeys at levels comparable to cocaine (0.05 mg/kg, i.v.). However, Deroche-Gamonet and colleagues (2002) reported that rats did not learn to self-administer modafinil (0.03-1.7 mg/kg, i.v.) over an 11-day period of acquisition. Furthermore in the latter study, modafinil (32-128 mg/kg, i.p.) did not alter (i.e., increase or decrease) cocaine (0.8 mg/kg, i.v.) self-administration, responding for cocaine self-administration under a progressive ratio schedule (a measure of reinforcer strength), or reinstatement of cocaine self-administration following extinction (a measure of relapse). Deroche-Gamonet and colleagues

(2002) also found that modafinil does not elicit a preference in the place preference procedure that measure the conditioned rewarding properties of abused drugs.

In the drug discrimination procedure, in which animals are trained to distinguish between injection of drug or placebo for delivery of a reinforcer (e.g., food pellet). Animals can learn to discriminate between cocaine or amphetamines and vehicle administration (Gold & Balster, 1996; Dopheide et al., 2007), indicating that these drugs induce a reliable interoceptive state; however, it has not been reported if modafinil could serve as a similar stimulus in animals. In tests with amphetamine and cocaine, modafinil produces a state similar to and augments the discriminative stimulus properties of the more-potent stimulants (Gold & Balster, 1996; Dopheide et al., 2007).

Presently, it is difficult to make any definitive conclusion about the addictive potential of modafinil from animal research. It is not clear whether modafinil is self-administered, which would indicate an abuse potential in humans, although the lack of modafinil-induced place preference and studies from human subjects suggests that an abuse potential should be a concern, but a lower risk than other stimulants. There is little or no animal research on repeated (e.g., chronic) modafinil treatment, which would be important to understand dependence. The findings from drug discrimination studies, as well as studies with humans, suggest that modafinil could be used as a substitution or replacement therapy for cocaine abuse or dependence.

Summary

Modafinil is pharmacologically active in animal models of human psychopathologies. It produces behavioral activation, but it is less potent than other stimulants. Consistent with its primary clinical applications, modafinil produces increased wakefulness and arousal in animals and improves performance on some learning, memory and cognition tasks. Regarding addiction, animal research is controversial at this point, although it appears that modafinil has reinforcing properties, albeit these are weak properties. Furthermore, modafinil does alter the behavioral properties of the other, stronger stimulants.

Modafinil's Mechanism of Action

Despite the widespread use of modafinil for its approved and off-label purposes, its mechanism of action in brain is unclear. No drug interacts with only a single target in the nervous system (e.g., selective serotonin reuptake inhibitor [SSRI] antidepressants bind to nicotinic acetylcholine receptors), but modafinil appears to have a very multifaceted profile. It is critical to evaluate and determine how modafinil works to both maximize its effectiveness and reduce maladaptive side effects, and to better understand its various treatment applications. As detailed below, various neurotransmitter systems (e.g., α_1 norepinephrine, serotonin (5-HT), amino acid, dopamine and orexin receptors, and dopamine transporters [DAT]) have been implicated in its actions through 20 years of research on the drug.

Adrenergic Receptors

α_1 norepinephrine receptors (adrenoceptors) have long been known to be involved in the regulation of motor activity and movement, possibly through increasing central dopamine transmission. Initial modafinil studies focused on a hypothesis that modafinil increased locomotor activity through the stimulation of α_1 adrenoceptors, most likely within areas involved in vigilance and arousal, such as hypothalamic regions (Duteil et al., 1990; Mignot, Nishino, Guilleminault, & Dement, 1994; Stone, Cotecchia, Lin, & Quartermain, 2002). Modafinil-induced increases in both motor activity in mice (4-256 mg/kg, i.p. or p.o.) and awakening (32-128 mg/kg, p.o.) in monkeys were minimized by central α_1 adrenoceptor antagonists, such as prazosin, but not by α_2 adrenoreceptor antagonists (Duteil et al., 1990). Various selective α_1 adrenoreceptor antagonists have been shown to attenuate modafinil (20 and 40 mg/kg, i.p.)-induced behavioral activation in mice and a diminished behavioral response to modafinil was observed in α_{1B} adrenoceptor knockout mice (Stone et al., 2002). Furthermore, α_1 adrenoceptor antagonists partially reversed modafinil-induced induced wakefulness in monkeys (16-64 mg/kg, p.o.; Hermant et al., 1991) and cats (1-5 mg/kg, p.o.; Lin et al., 1992).

Despite these initial findings, the current consensus in the literature is that modafinil does not work exclusively through α_1 adrenoceptors. Modafinil (≤ 10 μM) does not have good affinity for α_1 adrenoceptors, as measured by

[^{3}H]prazosin radioligand binding (Mignot et al., 1994). Modafinil (128 mg/kg, i.p.) failed to inhibit the firing rate of locus coeruleus noradrenergic neurons (Akaoka, Roussel, Lin, Chouvet, & Jouvet, 1991) and failed to decrease catechol oxidation peak height as measured by voltammetry in the mouse caudate nucleus and rat striatum or nucleus accumbens, indicating no activity to alter norepinephrine levels (Duteil et al., 1990).

Amino Acid Receptors

Noradrenaline exerts an excitatory action on gamma-aminobutyric (GABA) neurons via activation of α_1 adrenoceptors. If modafinil acts as a direct or indirect agonist of α_1 adrenoceptors, an increase in GABA release should be observed with the drug, which would indicate that the effects of modafinil may be partially modulated through GABA. Interestingly, however, modafinil (3-30 mg/kg, s.c.) reduced GABA release in the cortex, as measured via gas chromatography-mass spectrometry, the opposite of what would be expected of an α_1 adrenoreceptor agonist (Tanganelli et al., 1995). These findings were supported by microdialysis studies (Ferraro et al., 1996a; Ferraro et al., 1999), which found modafinil reduced levels of GABA, and also increased levels of glutamate, in the medial preoptic area and the posterior hypothalamus of the awake rat. Overall, these findings indicate that modafinil alters GABA neurotransmission, although, the modafinil-induced regulation is not direct. As examined via *in vivo* and *in vitro* methods, modafinil (100 mg/kg, i.p., and 10-1000 μM, respectively) had no effect on the synthesis of either GABA or glutamate in the rat hypothalamus (Perez et al., 1999). Moreover, as addressed below, the decrease in GABA release in the cerebral cortex, nucleus accumbens, medial preoptic area, and posterior hypothalamus may be mediated by other neurotransmitters, such as 5-HT (Tanganelli et al., 1995).

5-HT Receptors

The inhibitory control of GABAergic transmission by modafinil was partially or fully counteracted by pretreatment with various 5-HT receptor antagonists (Ferraro et al., 1996a; Tanganelli et al., 1995), suggesting that an increase in 5-HT activity is partially responsible for modafinil's effects. A series of studies by Ferraro and colleagues (2000; 2001; 2002; 2005) investigated further modafinil's influence on 5-HT activity. First, modafinil enhanced 5-HT transmission in the cerebral cortex of the awake rat (Ferraro et al., 2000). Unlike the 5-HT agonist *dl*-fenfluramine, and the SSRI fluoxetine, modafinil did not increase [^{3}H]5-HT release from rat cortical *synaptosomes*, but it did increase [^{3}H]5-HT release from preloaded rat cortical *slices* (Ferraro et al., 2000; Ferraro et al., 2001). The dichotomy between slices and synaptosomes suggests a presynaptic 5-HT influence, as intact presynaptic terminals are present in slices, but not in synaptosomes. Supporting the role for presynaptic 5-HT axon terminals, modafinil's influence on 5-HT in cortical slices became stronger in the presence of the SSRI paroxetine, but not in the presence of *dl*-fenfluramine, which seemed to block modafinil from acting presynaptically (Ferraro et al., 2001). Combined, these results suggest that modafinil does influence 5-HT release, but this ability requires interaction with intact 5-HT axon terminals.

The Ferraro group also used dual-probe microdialysis to determine the interaction of modafinil (3 mg/kg, i.p.) with the SSRI fluoxetine and imipramine (dual inhibitor of both norepinephrine and 5-HT uptake) on 5-HT levels in the rat dorsal raphe and prefrontal cortex (Ferraro et al., 2005). At low doses, modafinil further enhanced the increase in 5-HT levels seen with both fluoxetine and imipramine in the prefrontal cortex and enhanced the increase in 5-HT levels seen with fluoxetine in the raphe nucleus. However, by itself, modafinil was not effective in increasing 5-HT levels in either brain region. These findings are consistent with *in vivo* microdialysis findings in which modafinil enhanced extracellular 5-HT levels primarily in the frontal cortex (important for arousal) and the dorsal raphe (important for the regulation of REM sleep) but not in the medial preoptic area and the posterior hypothalamus (Ferraro et al., 2002). This indicates that modafinil's 5-HT effects are localized in regions important for maintaining the sleep/wake cycle. For example, the firing activity of 5-HT neurons in the dorsal raphe nucleus is highest in the waking state and decreases during sleep (see Ferraro et al., 2002). By enhancing 5-HT transmission in this brain region, modafinil may promote vigilance and arousal.

Orexin Receptors

Various studies also have linked the stimulant effects of modafinil to orexin receptors in hypothalamic pathways involved in the regulation of sleep and wakefulness. Scammell and colleagues (2000) correlated the wake-promoting effects of modafinil (75, 150, 300 mg/kg, i.p.) with patterns of neuronal activation in rats. Aside from promoting wakefulness, modafinil (75 and 150 mg, i.p.) strongly induced the transcription factor c-Fos, which increases when awake, in many brain regions (see Sagar, Sharp, & Curran, 1988). Importantly, an increase of c-Fos was found in orexin neurons in the perifornical area of the hypothalamus, a cell group implicated in maintaining wakefulness (Scammell et al., 2000). In supporting immunohistochemistry studies, modafinil again strongly induced the expression of c-Fos in hypothalamic and connected basal forebrain regions in the cat (Lin et al., 1992) and in rats (Engber et al., 1998). Together, these studies suggest that modafinil's wake-promoting effects come from activation of pathways of orexin neurons in the hypothalamus or perhaps from downstream activation of the connected basal forebrain.

Contrary to these findings, others have found that modafinil (10, 30, and 100 mg/kg, i.p.) produced similar patterns of neuronal and behavioral activation in both orexin-null and wild-type mice, as indicated by c-Fos immunohistochemistry, electroencephalograph, and various measures of wakefulness (Willie et al., 2005). In fact, contrary to what one would expect in a drug that worked via orexin receptor activation, modafinil produced a greater increase in wake time in orexin-null mice than in the wild-type mice. In this same study, modafinil partly compensated for attention deficits in the orexin-null mice. These findings suggest that it is not modafinil's wake-promoting effects, but perhaps attention/alerting effects, that result from the activation of orexin neurons (Willie et al., 2005).

While orexin's role is still unclear, the pattern of activation described may explain why modafinil is a stimulant, like amphetamine, but is devoid of amphetamine-like rewarding effects. Modafinil strongly induced the expression of c-Fos in hypothalamic and basal forebrain regions in the cat (Lin et al., 1992) and in rats (Engber et al., 1998) while amphetamine induced greater c-Fos in dopamine-responsive areas, such as the striatum (Lin et al., 1992). Perhaps this pattern of activation explains why modafinil does not have the dopamine-related addictive potential of amphetamine-like compounds.

Dopamine Transporters

Amphetamines are extremely potent and efficacious at increasing synaptic dopamine levels, which they achieve via functioning as a DAT substrate (Sulzer, Sonders, Poulsen, & Galli, 2005). Considering modafinil's amphetamine-like properties and its potential as an amphetamine and cocaine addiction treatment, the recent focus in the modafinil neuropharmacology literature has been its ability to alter dopamine levels, possibly through an interaction with DAT.

Several reports indicate that *in vitro* and *in vivo* modafinil elevates extracellular dopamine levels in brain. Ferraro and colleagues observed that modafinil increased dopamine levels in the rat nucleus accumbens via GABAergic mechanisms (Ferraro et al., 1996b; Ferraro et al., 1999). Supporting these findings, equipotent wake-promoting modafinil (5 mg/kg, i.v.) or amphetamine (0.1 mg/kg, i.v.) doses produced similar increases in striatal extracellular dopamine concentrations in narcoleptic animals (Nishino, Mao, Sampathkumaran, & Shelton, 1998). Administration of a wake-inducing modafinil (10 μg/5 μl) dose into the cerebral ventricles of rats resulted in increased dopamine levels in nucleus acumbens (Murillo-Rodriguez, Haro, Palomero-Rivero, Millan-Aldaco, & Drucker-Colin, 2007). Finally, in studies conducted in our laboratory, modafinil (100-300 μM) evoked [^{3}H]dopamine release from preloaded rat striatal slices in a concentration-dependent manner (Dopheide et al., 2007).

Several lines of evidence suggest that modafinil elevates dopamine levels in brain by altering DAT activity as an inhibitor or substrate for the transporter. Mignot and colleagues (1994) found that high concentrations of modafinil (>10 μM) inhibit neuronal dopamine uptake in rat brain, but did not bind to 5-HT, GABA, dopamine or glutamate receptors, calcium or potassium ion channels, or second messenger systems, suggesting that modafinil inhibited dopamine uptake by blocking DAT. The findings by Mignot and colleagues (1994) recently were supported by research where modafinil (~4-10 μM) inhibited [^{3}H]dopamine uptake in rat brain and blocked the DAT-mediated release of a transporter substrate (Zolkowska et al., 2009). In our laboratory (Dopheide et al., 2007), modafinil (100 μM)-evoked [^{3}H]dopamine release from preloaded rat striatal slices was attenuated by an excess concentration of the DAT inhibitor nomifensine. Positron emission tomography (PET) studies in monkeys and humans also indicate that modafinil binds to DAT. Modafinil (5 mg/kg, i.v.) inhibited the binding of DAT-selective radioligands in rhesus monkeys (Madras et al., 2006) and modafinil (200-400 mg, p.o.) prevented the binding of the radiolabeled cocaine, a DAT inhibitor, in humans (Volkow et al., 2009).

A functional role for DAT in modafinil's effects was supported in research with DAT knockout mice by Wisor and colleagues (2001). Deletion of the DAT gene increased wakefulness. As would be expected, both wild-type and DAT knock-out mice were equally sensitive to the wake-promoting effects of caffeine, a stimulant for which no direct action of the DAT has been reported; the wake-promoting effects of modafinil, methamphetamine, and known DAT inhibitors seen in wild-type mice were absent in the DAT knockout mice.

Alternatively or in addition to an interaction with DAT, modafinil could elevate dopamine levels via an interaction with D_1 and D_2 dopamine receptors (Young, 2009). Qu and colleagues (2008) demonstrated that a D_1 and a D_2 dopamine receptor antagonist blocked modafinil (22.5-45 mg/kg, i.p.)-induced arousal. Modafinil-induced arousal also was diminished in D_2 dopamine receptor knockout mice, and in knockout mice treated with a D_1 dopamine receptor antagonist.

Despite these findings supporting a role for dopamine, , other researchers suggest that modafinil's effects do not involve the catecholamine. Electrophysiological studies using extracellular recordings have shown that modafinil does not modify dopamine neuron firing rates in the ventral tegmental area or the substantia nigra in rats (Akaoka et al., 1991). Also, tyrosine hydroxylase inhibition, which would deplete intracellular dopamine levels, does not affect modafinil-induced, hyperlocomotion. These observations are in accordance with *in vivo* voltammetry studies performed by De Sereville and colleagues (1994) indicating that modafinil does not increase striatal extracellular levels of DA nor the DA metabolite, DOPAC, in anesthetized mice, whereas amphetamine and methylphenidate do increase these levels.

Summary

Early neurochemical findings suggested that modafinil's wake-promoting effects are dependent on α_1 adrenoceptor activation; however, opposite of what would be expected of an α_1 adrenoceptor agonist, modafinil inhibits (rather than increases) GABA release, especially in hypothalamic regions important for maintaining wakefulness. Interestingly, modafinil's inhibition of GABAergic transmission is mediated by 5-HT receptors, suggesting that an increased activity at presynaptic 5-HT axon terminals is at least partially responsible for modafinil's wake-promoting effects. However, research also suggests that modafinil's wake promoting actions do require dopaminergic activation via the DAT. Modafinil elevates dopamine levels via inhibition or reversal of DAT or via D_1 and D_2 dopamine receptors. The abuse and dependence liability of amphetamines are related to their ability to elevate dopamine levels, yet modafinil has a low abuse potential in humans and in animals. Modafinil's unique pattern of activation tends to be localized in orexin receptors in hypothalamic pathways (Engber et al., 1998;

Scammell et al., 2000), which may explain why it does not have similar abuse potential to stronger stimulants.

Conclusion

The above clinical, behavioral, and neurochemical data on modafinil show that modafinil is an effective wake-promoting agent that may prove to be a helpful treatment for a wide variety of sleep and mood disorders as well as mild cognitive impairment. While the research suggests that it does not have the addictive potential of typical stimulants, animal research suggests that it may enhance the incentive value of stronger stimulants. As for the mechanism of action of modafinil, the current literature suggests that many neurotransmitter systems are at work in producing modafinil's wake-promoting, mood-enhancing, and cognitive-enhancing effects.

Acknowledgment

The authors appreciate the contributions of Todd R. Schachtman (Department of Psychological Sciences, University of Missouri) and Russell E. Morgan (Department of Psychology, Western Illinois University) in this research line. Although we have not received funding from Cephalon and this chapter was not reviewed by Cephalon, we appreciate comments from and discussion with Dean Juge (Medical Science Liason, Cephalon) over the course of our research with modafinil.

References

Akaoka, H., Roussel, B., Lin, J. S., Chouvet, G. & Jouvet, M. (1991). Effect of modafinil and amphetamine on the rat catecholaminergic neuron activity. *Neurosci.Lett.*, *123*, 20-22.

Anderson, A. L., Reid, M. S., Li, S. H., Holmes, T., Shemanski, L., Slee, A., et al. (2009). Modafinil for the treatment of cocaine dependence. *Drug Alcohol Depend.*

Ballon, J. S. & Feifel, D. (2006). A systematic review of modafinil: Potential clinical uses and mechanisms of action. *J.Clin.Psychiatry*, *67*, 554-566.

Batejat, D. M. & Lagarde, D. P. (1999). Naps and modafinil as countermeasures for the effects of sleep deprivation on cognitive performance. *Aviat.Space Environ.Med.*, *70*, 493-498.

Beracochea, D., Cagnard, B., Celerier, A., le, M. J., Peres, M. & Pierard, C. (2001). First evidence of a delay-dependent working memory-enhancing effect of modafinil in mice. *Neuroreport*, *12*, 375-378.

Beracochea, D., Celerier, A., Borde, N., Valleau, M., Peres, M. & Pierard, C. (2002). Improvement of learning processes following chronic systemic administration of modafinil in mice. *Pharmacol.Biochem.Behav.*, *73*, 723-728.

Beracochea, D., Celerier, A., Peres, M. & Pierard, C. (2003). Enhancement of learning processes following an acute modafinil injection in mice. *Pharmacol.Biochem.Behav.*, *76*, 473-479.

Billiard, M. (2008). Narcolepsy: current treatment options and future approaches. *Neuropsychiatr.Dis.Treat.*, *4*, 557-566.

Billiard, M., Besset, A., Montplaisir, J., Laffont, F., Goldenberg, F., Weill, J. S. et al. (1994). Modafinil: a double-blind multicentric study. *Sleep*, *17*, S107-S112.

Bittencourt, L. R., Lucchesi, L. M., Rueda, A. D., Garbuio, S. A., Palombini, L. O., Guilleminault, C., et al. (2008). Placebo and modafinil effect on sleepiness in obstructive sleep apnea. *Prog.Neuropsychopharmacol. Biol.Psychiatry*, *32*, 552-559.

Black, J. E. & Hirshkowitz, M. (2005). Modafinil for treatment of residual excessive sleepiness in nasal continuous positive airway pressure-treated obstructive sleep apnea/hypopnea syndrome. *Sleep*, *28*, 464-471.

Broughton, R. J., Fleming, J. A., George, C. F., Hill, J. D., Kryger, M. H., Moldofsky, H., et al. (1997). Randomized, double-blind, placebo-controlled crossover trial of modafinil in the treatment of excessive daytime sleepiness in narcolepsy. *Neurology*, *49*, 444-451.

Caldwell, J. A. Jr., Caldwell, J. L., Smythe, N. K. III & Hall, K. K. (2000). A double-blind, placebo-controlled investigation of the efficacy of modafinil for sustaining the alertness and performance of aviators: a helicopter simulator study. *Psychopharmacology (Berl)*, *150*, 272-282.

Chapotot, F., Pigeau, R., Canini, F., Bourdon, L. & Buguet, A. (2003). Distinctive effects of modafinil and d-amphetamine on the homeostatic and circadian modulation of the human waking EEG. *Psychopharmacology (Berl), 166*, 127-138.

Czeisler, C. A., Walsh, J. K., Roth, T., Hughes, R. J., Wright, K. P., Kingsbury, L., et al. (2005). Modafinil for excessive sleepiness associated with shift-work sleep disorder. *N.Engl.J.Med., 353*, 476-486.

Dackis, C. A., Kampman, K. M., Lynch, K. G., Pettinati, H. M. & O'Brien, C. P. (2005). A double-blind, placebo-controlled trial of modafinil for cocaine dependence. *Neuropsychopharmacology, 30*, 205-211.

Dackis, C. A., Lynch, K. G., Yu, E., Samaha, F. F., Kampman, K. M., Cornish, J. W., et al. (2003). Modafinil and cocaine: a double-blind, placebo-controlled drug interaction study. *Drug Alcohol Depend., 70*, 29-37.

De Sereville, J. E., Boer, C., Rambert, F. A. & Duteil, J. (1994). Lack of pre-synaptic dopaminergic involvement in modafinil activity in anaesthetized mice: in vivo voltammetry studies. *Neuropharmacology, 33*, 755-761.

Deroche-Gamonet, V., Darnaudery, M., Bruins-Slot, L., Piat, F., Le, M. M. & Piazza, P. V. (2002). Study of the addictive potential of modafinil in naive and cocaine-experienced rats. *Psychopharmacology (Berl), 161*, 387-395.

Dopheide, M. M., Morgan, R. E., Rodvelt, K. R., Schachtman, T. R. & Miller, D. K. (2007). Modafinil evokes striatal [^{3}H]dopamine release and alters the subjective properties of stimulants. *Eur.J.Pharmacol., 568*, 112-123.

Duteil, J., Rambert, F. A., Pessonnier, J., Hermant, J. F., Gombert, R. & Assous, E. (1990). Central α_1-adrenergic stimulation in relation to the behaviour stimulating effect of modafinil; studies with experimental animals. *Eur.J.Pharmacol., 180*, 49-58.

Edgar, D. M. & Seidel, W. F. (1997). Modafinil induces wakefulness without intensifying motor activity or subsequent rebound hypersomnolence in the rat. *J.Pharmacol.Exp.Ther., 283*, 757-769.

Eliyahu, U., Berlin, S., Hadad, E., Heled, Y. & Moran, D. S. (2007). Psychostimulants and military operations. *Mil.Med., 172*, 383-387.

Engber, T. M., Koury, E. J., Dennis, S. A., Miller, M. S., Contreras, P. C. & Bhat, R. V. (1998). Differential patterns of regional c-Fos induction in the rat brain by amphetamine and the novel wakefulness-promoting agent modafinil. *Neurosci.Lett., 241*, 95-98.

Fava, M., Thase, M. E. & DeBattista, C. (2005). A multicenter, placebo-controlled study of modafinil augmentation in partial responders to selective serotonin reuptake inhibitors with persistent fatigue and sleepiness. *J.Clin.Psychiatry, 66*, 85-93.

Ferraro, L., Antonelli, T., Tanganelli, S., O'Connor, W. T., Perez, d. l. M., Mendez-Franco, J., et al. (1999). The vigilance promoting drug modafinil increases extracellular glutamate levels in the medial preoptic area and the posterior hypothalamus of the conscious rat: prevention by local GABAA receptor blockade. *Neuropsychopharmacology*, *20*, 346-356.

Ferraro, L., Fuxe, K., Agnati, L., Tanganelli, S., Tomasini, M. C. & Antonelli, T. (2005). Modafinil enhances the increase of extracellular serotonin levels induced by the antidepressant drugs fluoxetine and imipramine: a dual probe microdialysis study in awake rat. *Synapse*, *55*, 230-241.

Ferraro, L., Fuxe, K., Tanganelli, S., Fernandez, M., Rambert, F. A. & Antonelli, T. (2000). Amplification of cortical serotonin release: a further neurochemical action of the vigilance-promoting drug modafinil. *Neuropharmacology*, *39*, 1974-1983.

Ferraro, L., Fuxe, K., Tanganelli, S., Tomasini, M. C., Rambert, F. A. & Antonelli, T. (2002). Differential enhancement of dialysate serotonin levels in distinct brain regions of the awake rat by modafinil: possible relevance for wakefulness and depression. *J.Neurosci.Res.*, *68*, 107-112.

Ferraro, L., Tanganelli, S., Fuxe, K., Bebe, B. W., Tomasini, M. C., Rambert, F. A., et al. (2001). Modafinil does not affect serotonin efflux from rat frontal cortex synaptosomes: comparison with known serotonergic drugs. *Brain Res.*, *894*, 307-310.

Ferraro, L., Tanganelli, S., O'Connor, W. T., Antonelli, T., Rambert, F. & Fuxe, K. (1996a). The vigilance promoting drug modafinil decreases GABA release in the medial preoptic area and in the posterior hypothalamus of the awake rat: possible involvement of the serotonergic 5-HT_3 receptor. *Neurosci.Lett.*, *220*, 5-8.

Ferraro, L., Tanganelli, S., O'Connor, W. T., Antonelli, T., Rambert, F. & Fuxe, K. (1996b). The vigilance promoting drug modafinil increases dopamine release in the rat nucleus accumbens via the involvement of a local GABAergic mechanism. *Eur.J.Pharmacol.*, *306*, 33-39.

Gold, L. H. & Balster, R. L. (1996). Evaluation of the cocaine-like discriminative stimulus effects and reinforcing effects of modafinil. *Psychopharmacology (Berl)*, *126*, 286-292.

Gonon, F. (2009). The dopaminergic hypothesis of attention-deficit/ hyperactivity disorder needs re-examining. *Trends Neurosci.*, *32*, 2-8.

Hart, C. L., Haney, M., Vosburg, S. K., Rubin, E. & Foltin, R. W. (2008). Smoked cocaine self-administration is decreased by modafinil. *Neuropsychopharmacology*, *33*, 761-768.

Hermant, J. F., Rambert, F. A. & Duteil, J. (1991). Awakening properties of modafinil: effect on nocturnal activity in monkeys (*Macaca mulatta*) after acute and repeated administration. *Psychopharmacology (Berl), 103*, 28-32.

Kaufman, K. R., Menza, M. A. & Fitzsimmons, A. (2002). Modafinil monotherapy in depression. *Eur.Psychiatry, 17*, 167-169.

Kingshott, R. N., Vennelle, M., Coleman, E. L., Engleman, H. M., Mackay, T. W. & Douglas, N. J. (2001). Randomized, double-blind, placebo-controlled crossover trial of modafinil in the treatment of residual excessive daytime sleepiness in the sleep apnea/hypopnea syndrome. *Am.J.Respir.Crit Care Med., 163*, 918-923.

Kumar, R. (2008). Approved and investigational uses of modafinil : an evidence-based review. *Drugs, 68*, 1803-1839.

Lagarde, D. & Milhaud, C. (1990). Electroencephalographic effects of modafinil, an alpha-1-adrenergic psychostimulant, on the sleep of rhesus monkeys. *Sleep, 13*, 441-448.

Lam, J. Y., Freeman, M. K. & Cates, M. E. (2007). Modafinil augmentation for residual symptoms of fatigue in patients with a partial response to antidepressants. *Ann.Pharmacother., 41*, 1005-1012.

Lankford, D. A. (2008). Armodafinil: a new treatment for excessive sleepiness. *Expert.Opin.Investig.Drugs, 17*, 565-573.

Liepert, J., Allstadt-Schmitz, J. & Weiller, C. (2004). Motor excitability and motor behaviour after modafinil ingestion--a double-blind placebo-controlled cross-over trial. *J.Neural Transm., 111*, 703-711.

Lin, J. S., Roussel, B., Akaoka, H., Fort, P., Debilly, G. & Jouvet, M. (1992). Role of catecholamines in the modafinil and amphetamine induced wakefulness, a comparative pharmacological study in the cat. *Brain Res., 591*, 319-326.

Lindsay, S. E., Gudelsky, G. A. & Heaton, P. C. (2006). Use of modafinil for the treatment of attention deficit/hyperactivity disorder. *Ann.Pharmacother., 40*, 1829-1833.

Madras, B. K., Xie, Z., Lin, Z., Jassen, A., Panas, H., Lynch, L., et al. (2006). Modafinil occupies dopamine and norepinephrine transporters in vivo and modulates the transporters and trace amine activity in vitro. *J.Pharmacol.Exp.Ther., 319*, 561-569.

Markovitz, P. J. & Wagner, S. (2003). An open-label trial of modafinil augmentation in patients with partial response to antidepressant therapy. *J.Clin.Psychopharmacol., 23*, 207-209.

Menza, M. A., Kaufman, K. R. & Castellanos, A. (2000). Modafinil augmentation of antidepressant treatment in depression. *J.Clin.Psychiatry*, *61*, 378-381.

Mignot, E., Nishino, S., Guilleminault, C. & Dement, W. C. (1994). Modafinil binds to the dopamine uptake carrier site with low affinity. *Sleep*, *17*, 436-437.

Minzenberg, M. J. & Carter, C. S. (2008). Modafinil: a review of neurochemical actions and effects on cognition. *Neuropsychopharmacology*, *33*, 1477-1502.

Morgan, R. E., Crowley, J. M., Smith, R. H., LaRoche, R. B. & Dopheide, M. M. (2007). Modafinil improves attention, inhibitory control, and reaction time in healthy, middle-aged rats. *Pharmacol.Biochem.Behav.*, *86*, 531-541.

Muller, U., Steffenhagen, N., Regenthal, R. & Bublak, P. (2004). Effects of modafinil on working memory processes in humans. *Psychopharmacology (Berl)*, *177*, 161-169.

Murillo-Rodriguez, E., Haro, R., Palomero-Rivero, M., Millan-Aldaco, D. & Drucker-Colin, R. (2007). Modafinil enhances extracellular levels of dopamine in the nucleus accumbens and increases wakefulness in rats. *Behav.Brain Res.*, *176*, 353-357.

Nishino, S., Mao, J., Sampathkumaran, R. & Shelton, J. (1998). Increased dopaminergic transmission mediates the wake-promoting effects of CNS stimulants. *Sleep Res.Online.*, *1*, 49-61.

Orr, K. & Taylor, D. (2007). Psychostimulants in the treatment of depression : a review of the evidence. *CNS.Drugs*, *21*, 239-257.

Pack, A. I., Black, J. E., Schwartz, J. R. & Matheson, J. K. (2001). Modafinil as adjunct therapy for daytime sleepiness in obstructive sleep apnea. *Am.J.Respir.Crit Care Med.*, *164*, 1675-1681.

Perez, d. l. M., Aguilar-Garcia, A., Ramon-Frias, T., Ramirez-Ramirez, R., Mendez-Franco, J., Rambert, F. et al. (1999). Effects of the vigilance promoting drug modafinil on the synthesis of GABA and glutamate in slices of rat hypothalamus. *Neurosci.Lett.*, *259*, 181-185.

Qu, W. M., Huang, Z. L., Xu, X. H., Matsumoto, N. & Urade, Y. (2008). Dopaminergic D_1 and D_2 receptors are essential for the arousal effect of modafinil. *J.Neurosci.*, *28*, 8462-8469.

Randall, D. C., Shneerson, J. M., Plaha, K. K. & File, S. E. (2003). Modafinil affects mood, but not cognitive function, in healthy young volunteers. *Hum.Psychopharmacol.*, *18*, 163-173.

Randomized trial of modafinil as a treatment for the excessive daytime somnolence of narcolepsy: US Modafinil in Narcolepsy Multicenter Study Group (2000). *Neurology*, *54*, 1166-1175.

Randomized trial of modafinil for the treatment of pathological somnolence in narcolepsy. US Modafinil in Narcolepsy Multicenter Study Group (1998). *Ann.Neurol.*, *43*, 88-97.

Rosenthal, M. H. & Bryant, S. L. (2004). Benefits of adjunct modafinil in an open-label, pilot study in patients with schizophrenia. *Clin.Neuropharmacol.*, *27*, 38-43.

Rugino, T. A. & Copley, T. C. (2001). Effects of modafinil in children with attention-deficit/hyperactivity disorder: an open-label study. *J.Am.Acad.Child Adolesc.Psychiatry*, *40*, 230-235.

Rugino, T. A. & Samsock, T. C. (2003). Modafinil in children with attention-deficit hyperactivity disorder. *Pediatr.Neurol.*, *29*, 136-142.

Rush, C. R., Kelly, T. H., Hays, L. R. & Wooten, A. F. (2002). Discriminative-stimulus effects of modafinil in cocaine-trained humans. *Drug Alcohol Depend.*, *67*, 311-322.

Rush, C. R., Kelly, T. H., Hays, L. R., Baker, R. W. & Wooten, A. F. (2002). Acute behavioral and physiological effects of modafinil in drug abusers. *Behav.Pharmacol.*, *13*, 105-115.

Sagar, S. M., Sharp, F. R. & Curran, T. (1988). Expression of c-fos protein in brain: metabolic mapping at the cellular level. *Science*, *240*, 1328-1331.

Scammell, T. E., Estabrooke, I. V., McCarthy, M. T., Chemelli, R. M., Yanagisawa, M., Miller, M. S., et al. (2000). Hypothalamic arousal regions are activated during modafinil-induced wakefulness. *J.Neurosci.*, *20*, 8620-8628.

Schnoll, R. A., Wileyto, E. P., Pinto, A., Leone, F., Gariti, P., Siegel, S., et al. (2008). A placebo-controlled trial of modafinil for nicotine dependence. *Drug Alcohol Depend.*, *98*, 86-93.

Schwartz, J. R. (2005). Modafinil: new indications for wake promotion. *Expert.Opin.Pharmacother.*, *6*, 115-129.

Schwartz, J. R., Feldman, N. T. & Bogan, R. K. (2005). Dose effects of modafinil in sustaining wakefulness in narcolepsy patients with residual evening sleepiness. *J.Neuropsychiatry Clin.Neurosci.*, *17*, 405-412.

Sevy, S., Rosenthal, M. H., Alvir, J., Meyer, S., Visweswaraiah, H., Gunduz-Bruce, H., et al. (2005). Double-blind, placebo-controlled study of modafinil for fatigue and cognition in schizophrenia patients treated with psychotropic medications. *J.Clin.Psychiatry*, *66*, 839-843.

Shearer, J., Darke, S., Rodgers, C., Slade, T., van, B., I, Lewis, J., et al. (2009). A double-blind, placebo-controlled trial of modafinil (200 mg/day) for methamphetamine dependence. *Addiction*, *104*, 224-233.

Shelton, J., Nishino, S., Vaught, J., Dement, W. C. & Mignot, E. (1995). Comparative effects of modafinil and amphetamine on daytime sleepiness and cataplexy of narcoleptic dogs. *Sleep*, *18*, 817-826.

Simon, P., Hemet, C. & Costentin, J. (1996). Analysis of stimulant locomotor effects of modafinil in various strains of mice and rats. *Fundam.Clin.Pharmacol.*, *10*, 431-435.

Simon, P., Panissaud, C. & Costentin, J. (1994). The stimulant effect of modafinil on wakefulness is not associated with an increase in anxiety in mice. A comparison with dexamphetamine. *Psychopharmacology (Berl)*, *114*, 597-600.

Sofuoglu, M. & Kosten, T. R. (2006). Emerging pharmacological strategies in the fight against cocaine addiction. *Expert.Opin.Emerg.Drugs*, *11*, 91-98.

Spiller, H. A., Borys, D., Griffith, J. R., Klein-Schwartz, W., Aleguas, A., Sollee, D., et al. (2009). Toxicity from modafinil ingestion. *Clin.Toxicol.(Phila)*, *47*, 153-156.

Stone, E. A., Cotecchia, S., Lin, Y. & Quartermain, D. (2002). Role of brain α_{1B}-adrenoceptors in modafinil-induced behavioral activity. *Synapse*, *46*, 269-270.

Stoops, W. W., Lile, J. A., Fillmore, M. T., Glaser, P. E. & Rush, C. R. (2005). Reinforcing effects of modafinil: influence of dose and behavioral demands following drug administration. *Psychopharmacology (Berl)*, *182*, 186-193.

Sulzer, D., Sonders, M. S., Poulsen, N. W. & Galli, A. (2005). Mechanism of neurotransmitter release by amphetamines: A review. *Progress in Neurobiology*, *75*, 406-433.

Tanganelli, S., Perez, d. l. M., Ferraro, L., Mendez-Franco, J., Beani, L., Rambert, F. A., et al. (1995). Modafinil and cortical gamma-aminobutyric acid outflow. Modulation by 5-hydroxytryptamine neurotoxins. *Eur.J.Pharmacol.*, *273*, 63-71.

Taylor, F. B. & Russo, J. (2000). Efficacy of modafinil compared to dextroamphetamine for the treatment of attention deficit hyperactivity disorder in adults. *J.Child Adolesc.Psychopharmacol.*, *10*, 311-320.

Teitelman, E. (2001). Off-label uses of modafinil. *Am.J.Psychiatry*, *158*, 1341.

Touret, M., Sallanon-Moulin, M. & Jouvet, M. (1995). Awakening properties of modafinil without paradoxical sleep rebound: comparative study with amphetamine in the rat. *Neurosci.Lett.*, *189*, 43-46.

Turner, D. C., Clark, L., Pomarol-Clotet, E., McKenna, P., Robbins, T. W. & Sahakian, B. J. (2004). Modafinil improves cognition and attentional set shifting in patients with chronic schizophrenia. *Neuropsychopharmacology*, *29*, 1363-1373.

Turner, D. C., Robbins, T. W., Clark, L., Aron, A. R., Dowson, J. & Sahakian, B. J. (2003). Cognitive enhancing effects of modafinil in healthy volunteers. *Psychopharmacology (Berl)*, *165*, 260-269.

Vocci, F. J. & Elkashef, A. (2005). Pharmacotherapy and other treatments for cocaine abuse and dependence. *Curr.Opin.Psychiatry*, *18*, 265-270.

Volkow, N. D., Fowler, J. S., Logan, J., Alexoff, D., Zhu, W., Telang, F., et al. (2009). Effects of modafinil on dopamine and dopamine transporters in the male human brain: clinical implications. *JAMA*, *301*, 1148-1154.

Vorspan, F., Warot, D., Consoli, A., Cohen, D. & Mazet, P. (2005). Mania in a boy treated with modafinil for narcolepsy. *Am.J.Psychiatry*, *162*, 813-814.

Walsh, J. K., Randazzo, A. C., Stone, K. L. & Schweitzer, P. K. (2004). Modafinil improves alertness, vigilance, and executive function during simulated night shifts. *Sleep*, *27*, 434-439.

Warot, D., Corruble, E., Payan, C., Weil, J. S. & Puech, A. J. (1993). Subjective effects of modafinil, a new central adrenergic stimulant in healthy volunteers: A comparison with amphetamine, caffeine and placebo. *European Psychiatry*, *8*, 201-208.

Waters, K. A., Burnham, K. E., O'connor, D., Dawson, G. R. & Dias, R. (2005). Assessment of modafinil on attentional processes in a five-choice serial reaction time test in the rat. *J.Psychopharmacol.*, *19*, 149-158.

Wesensten, N. J., Killgore, W. D. & Balkin, T. J. (2005). Performance and alertness effects of caffeine, dextroamphetamine, and modafinil during sleep deprivation. *J.Sleep Res.*, *14*, 255-266.

Willie, J. T., Renthal, W., Chemelli, R. M., Miller, M. S., Scammell, T. E., Yanagisawa, M., et al. (2005). Modafinil more effectively induces wakefulness in orexin-null mice than in wild-type littermates. *Neuroscience*, *130*, 983-995.

Wisor, J. P., Nishino, S., Sora, I., Uhl, G. H., Mignot, E. & Edgar, D. M. (2001). Dopaminergic role in stimulant-induced wakefulness. *J.Neurosci.*, *21*, 1787-1794.

Young, J. W. (2009). Dopamine D_1 and D_2 receptor family contributions to modafinil-induced wakefulness. *J.Neurosci.*, *29*, 2663-2665.

Zolkowska, D., Jain, R., Rothman, R. B., Partilla, J. S., Roth, B. L., Setola, V., et al. (2009). Evidence for the involvement of dopamine transporters in behavioral stimulant effects of modafinil. *J.Pharmacol.Exp.Ther.*, *329*, 738-746.

In: Nacrolepsy: Symptoms, Causes... ISBN: 978-1-60876-645-1
Editors: G. Santos et al. pp. 65-85

Chapter III

Lights and Pitfalls in the Diagnosis of Narcolepsy

Rocco Salvatore Calabrò, Giuseppe Gervasi, Donatella Imbesi and Placido Bramanti
IRCCS Centro Neurolesi "Bonino-Pulejo", Messina.

Abstract

Narcolepsy is a clinical syndrome defined by four symptoms: a compliant excessive sleepiness; a sudden bilateral loss of postural muscle tone or a sudden muscle weakness, often subsequent to an intense emotion (Cataplexy); sleep paralysis; hypnagogic hallucinations. The syndrome can be idiopathic or secondary to other medical condition (neurological diseases, other sleep disorders or drugs abuse). In the presence of pathognomonic clinical criteria, diagnosis is confirmed by video-polysomnography (vPSG), Multiple Sleep latency Test (MLST). The presence of HLA-DR2 and low hypocretin values in cerebrospinal fluid can support this diagnosis.

According to the International Classification of Sleep Disorders (ICSD-2v) we can distinguish Narcolepsy into two major groups: Narcolepsy with or without cataplexy.

The main difference between the two entities is the absence of typical cataplexy and the necessity in narcolepsy without cataplexy to confirm the clinical diagnosis by nocturnal vPSG followed by MSLT showing two or more sleep onset REM periods.

Narcolepsy with Cataplexy is often misdiagnosed as a psychiatric condition or as an epilepsy variant or other form of hypersomnia (i.e. sleep apnea syndrome, hypersomnia due to depression). When cataplexy is predominant, Narcolepsy can be misdiagnosed as syncope, drop attacks, atonic attacks or attacks of a histrionic nature. Instead when sleep paralysis and/or hypnagogic hallucinations are predominant symptoms, narcolepsy can be confounded for psychological/psychiatric disease, but also for other REM parasomnia.

Narcolepsy without cataplexy may overlap with idiopathic hypersomnia.

In conclusion a correct diagnosis of narcolepsy is important since this syndrome has a good outcome and, usually, improves with specific drugs (modafinil, sodium oxybate, SSRI, tricyclic antidepressants). Moreover, erroneous treatments due to a misdiagnosis can precipitate or exacerbate the symptoms of Narcolepsy.

Introduction

Narcolepsy is defined as “a sleep disorder of unknown etiology, which is characterized by excessive sleepiness that typically is associated with cataplexy and other REM sleep phenomena such as sleep paralysis and hypnagogic hallucinations”. Historically narcolepsy is one of the most studied sleep disorders. In 1880 Gèlineàu was the first author to describe this syndrome and coined the term narcolepsy to individuate a group of patient with excessive daytime sleepiness (EDS), sleep attacks and episodes of muscle weakness triggered by emotions.

In the following decades many authors worked hard to promote and improve a systematic classification of sleep disorders. In the International Classification of Sleep Disorders (ICSD) narcolepsy was well defined, but the final classification and approved diagnostic criteria of Narcolepsy were finally reviewed by the American Academy of Sleep Medicine in the ICSD 2nd version (ICSD-2v) [1,2]

Clinically narcolepsy is a syndrome characterized by four symptoms, often defined as narcoleptic “tetrad”:

1. compliant EDS;
2. sudden bilateral loss of postural muscle tone or a or sudden muscle weakness called “Cataplexy”, often subsequent to an intense emotion;
3. sleep paralysis;

4. hypnagogic (at sleep onset) or hypnopompic (at wake onset) hallucinations.

The *prevalence* of narcolepsy is about 0.05% in United States and Western Europe population, higher in Japan (0.18%) while lower in Israel (0.002%) [3]. The age of onset varies from the childhood to young adults, with a bimodal distribution including a large peak during the second decade (about 14-15 years) and a second smaller peak at about 35-36 years [4,5]

Narcolepsy can be distinguished into an idiopathic form and into a symptomatic form due to other medical condition (i.e. neurological or other sleep disorders, drugs abuse, etc).

E*tiopathogenesis* of the idiopathic narcolepsy is still unknown. The most recent hypothesis suggests that narcolepsy could be a neurodegenerative disorder with an autoimmune component triggering the onset of the disease in susceptible individuals [6]. This hypothesis supposes a self damage to the hypothalamic hypocretin (Hct) producing neurons. Hcts are excitatory neurotransmitters and modulators of central nervous system involving serotoninergic, histaminergic, dopaminergic, acetylcholinergic and more over pathways, with a vast array of functions, especially those involved in the regulation of sleep-wake cycle. [7,8].

Low dosage of Hct in cerebrospinal fluid has been shown to be specific for patients with HLA DR2 (especially DQB1*0602) positive narcolepsy with cataplexy and it is noted in the early stages of the disease [9]. However newer studies in the last 10 years show discordant results about familiarity of this disease: studies on the first-relatives of narcoleptic patients demonstrate an increasing risk (10-40 times higher than the general population) of developing the disease [10,11] while the twin studies report only a concordance of 25-31%, suggesting a major contribution of environmental factors [12,13]. Despite the association with a specific HLA gene (DQB1*0602), an autoimmune origin of narcolepsy remains controversial and an attempt to find the specific auto-antibody to these HLA genes has to date been unsuccessful [14].

Beside the autoimmune damage many environmental factors are documented to trigger or exacerbate symptoms of narcolepsy. The most frequent environmental factors involved in the development of narcolepsy are head trauma, sudden change in sleep/wake habits, psychological stress, pregnancy or various infections determining bilateral encephalitis [5,15-17].

Symptoms of narcolepsy can also be seen during the course of a neurological disease process. A recent review by Nishino has underlined the importance of the hypothalamus in symptomatic narcolepsy, cataplexy and hypersomnia. In particular, it seems that the common pathway through neurological diseases (i.e. head trauma, brain tumor, encephalitis, heredo-degenerative disorders, etc) acting in the development of symptomatic narcolepsy is the involvement of lateral hypothalamic area, where Hct producing neurons are present [18-20]

Diagnostic Criteria

Diagnosis of narcolepsy is based on clinical evaluation of the symptoms fulfilling the diagnostic criteria of the ICSD-2v [2] and it is classified into a form with cataplexy and a form without cataplexy, as shown in Table 1 and Table 2.

Table 1. ICSD-2 diagnostic criteria of narcolepsy with cataplexy.

A.	The patient has a complaint of excessive daytime sleepiness occurring almost daily for at least three months.
B.	A definite history of cataplexy, defined as sudden and transient episodes of loss of motor tone triggered by emotions is present.
C.	The diagnosis of narcolepsy with cataplexy should, whenever possible, be confirmed by nocturnal polysomnography followed by an MSLT; the mean sleep latency on MSLT is less than or equal to 8 min and two or more SOREMPs are observed following sufficient nocturnal sleep (minimum 6 h) during the night prior to the test. Alternatively, hypocretin-1 levels in the CSF are less than or equal to 110 pg/ml or one-third of mean normal values.
D.	The hypersomnia is not better explained by another sleep disorder or neurological disorder, mental disorder, medication use, or substance use disorder.

Clinical evaluation of narcolepsy may be difficult because it has a typical variable phenotype: the presence or absence of symptoms may vary during the course of the illness and, moreover, not all symptoms are present at the onset of the disease or in the same subject. Only about 10% of patients develop the full tetrad [6]. EDS and cataplexy are often the first appearing and also the more specific symptoms of the disease. Sleep paralysis and sleep-related hallucinations are present in about 50% of the narcoleptic patients, but also non narcoleptic persons can present these features. So EDS and cataplexy are also called cardinal symptoms as their presence is pathognomonic of narcolepsy, while sleep paralysis and sleep-related hallucinations are also called associated (or ancillary) features as their presence can corroborate but not are essential for the diagnosis.

The age of onset of idiopathic form is often in the childhood or young age (especially in the age range 10-25 years with a peak occurring at 14.7 years) and it typically shows all of the four symptoms. EDS is frequently noted as the first symptom of the disease in children, while patients over 60 years reported more often cataplexy as their initial symptom. Diagnosis of narcolepsy is harder especially in pediatric patients that slowly develop the symptoms and it could be easily misdiagnosed as behavioral disorders, malingering, epilepsy and/or other causes of hypersomnia. Many studies showed that children suffering of narcolepsy are referred to many physicians before the correct diagnosis is finally made. Moreover a recent study shows that only 38% of 77 narcoleptic patients received a correct diagnosis before the sleep specialist evaluation. Misdiagnosis results in a significant delay in treatment, with many patients labeled as lazy or "acting out". This is especially important in the adolescent age group as career decisions that have a lifetime impact are being made during this time [21,22].

Table 2. ICSD-2 diagnostic criteria of narcolepsy without cataplexy.

A.	The patient has a complaint of excessive daytime sleepiness occurring almost daily for at least three months.
B.	Typical cataplexy is not present, although doubtful or atypical cataplexy-like episodes may be reported.
C.	The diagnosis of narcolepsy without cataplexy must be confirmed by nocturnal polysomnography followed by an MSLT. In narcolepsy without cataplexy, the mean sleep latency on MSLT is less than or equal to 8 min and two or more SOREMPs are observed following sufficient nocturnal sleep (minimum 6 h) during the night prior to the test.
D.	The hypersomnia is not better explained by another sleep disorder, medical or neurological disorder, mental disorder, medication use, or substance use disorder.

Adulthood is usually the age of onset of secondary form, whereas a cause of the disease is most commonly identified. In contrast to the idiopathic form, symptomatic narcolepsy could not present with the complete diagnostic tetrad [6].

The general course of the disease is difficult to describe. The order in which symptoms appear varies. Sleepiness and cataplexy persist throughout life although they often improve after retirement, probably owning to better management of activities, daytime napping and adjustment of night-time sleep [4].

To confirm the diagnosis of narcolepsy, patients must undergo a night-time video-polysomnography (PSG) followed by a Multiple Sleep Latency Test (MSLT). The instrumental criteria are necessary especially for the diagnosis of narcolepsy without cataplexy. The aim of PSG is to eliminate other sleep disorders cause of daytime sleepiness and to assess whether the patient has had enough sleep (at least 6 hour) before the MSLT [4].

PSG might show an alteration of the regular sleep pattern: a reduced sleep latency (less than 10 minutes), in particular a reduced nocturnal REM-sleep latency (less than 60 minutes); an increased total REM-sleep time, with a fragmentation in REM-sleep and imperfect loss of muscle tone; an increased proportion of Stage 1; a reduced Slow Waves Sleep, with an its relative augmentation at the end of the night [1,2,4].

The aim of MSLT is to assess the EDS. A standard MSLT consists in five naps scheduled at 2-h intervals starting in the morning after the PSG. MSLT can demonstrate an average sleep latency less than 8 minutes and the presence of two or more sleep onset REM periods (SOREMPs) [2,4,23]. The American Sleep Disorders Association recommends that an MSLT should be performed for all patients suspected of narcolepsy [24]. However, the diagnostic values of MSLT has been recently questioned by some authors: first, approximately 15% of narcoleptic subjects do not have a diagnostic MSLT; second, a small number of patients with other sleep disorders (especially sleep related breathing disorders) may display a typical narcolepsy-like MSLT results [25]. For this reason, other polygraphic methods have been developed to measure EDS, such as the sleep latency in the Maintenance of Wakefulness Test, even if to date it is generally used to assess the effect of treatment with psychostimulants [15,26,27]

The diagnosis of narcolepsy can be moreover confirmed by the presence of a DR2 positivity at HLA typing and the reduced levels of Hct (less than 110 pg/ml) in the cerebrospinal fluid (CSF).

The association between narcolepsy and HLA genes was studied since 1984 when Juji and coworkers showed an association of 100% in Japanese narcoleptic people. A close association subsequently was confirmed in Europe and North America [14,28,29]. In the last years the amplification of the polymorphic exon of the HLA DQA and DQB gene by polymerase chain reaction has shown that all Caucasian narcoleptic patients have the same allele (DRB1*1501, DQA1*0102 and DQB1*0602). However, the most specific markers of a narcoleptic patient in a number of different ethnic groups studied to date is DQB1*0602 [30,31].

It was found that the large majority of patients (about 85-90%) with narcolepsy-cataplexy have low or undetectable Hct-1 ligand in their CSF [32]. Hct-1 deficiency is closely associated with the occurrence of cataplexy and HLA-DQ1*0602 genotype among narcoleptic subjects [33,34]. Low CSF Hct-1 appears to be a more specific test than the MSLT, although such low dosage is also seen in a few other neurological conditions (i.e. Guillain Barrè, Ma2 positive paraneoplastic syndrome) and about 10% of narcolepsy-cataplexy patients have normal CSF Hct-1 [15,30,35,36]. Since diagnosis is generally straight forwards in patient with cataplexy, CFS Hct-1 is only measured if the usual diagnostic procedures are not sufficient. These situations are: equivocal MSLT; patient unable to follow a correct MSLT (i.e. children or neurological or psychiatric patients); patient taking psychotropic medication. In these cases, lower CSF Hct-1 concentration than 110 ng/L or 30% of local normal values are highly indicative of idiopathic narcolepsy. Several researchers have found that the CSF Hct-1 concentration was almost always above 200 ng/L in controls or individuals with other sleep and neurological disorders [2,4,33,37].

Differential Diagnosis: Lights and Pitfalls

Narcolepsy can be confused with other forms of hypersomnolence, such as sleep apnea syndrome (SAS), idiopathic hypersomnia (IH), recurrent hypersomnia (RH), hypersomnia associated with depression and chronic sleep deprivation. All of these causes of hypersomnolence can determine a compliant EDS similar to narcolepsy. The presence of cataplexy is the key factor to single out narcolepsy from other causes of hypersomnia [4,15].

SAS is one of the major causes of daytime sleepiness, usually in middle-aged rather than young persons, and it can confound the MSLT evaluation. SAS is a common disorder, characterized by repetitive pharyngeal collapse during sleep. To restore pharyngeal patency, individuals have recurrent arousals from sleep, which lead to activation of sympathetic nervous system and fragmentation of sleep. This can lead to neurocognitive impairment, decreased quality of life, and increased risk of motor vehicle and occupational accidents. SAS is more frequent in male than female (about five to six-fold higher) as it is present from 20 to 24% of men and from 7 to 10% in female. Nasal continuous positive airway pressure is the most used treatment for SAS on the basis of improvements in clinical features

[38]. Asymptomatic sleep apnea can present with, but not linked to, narcolepsy. In cases where it is not clear if the two conditions are linked, especially when cataplexy is questionable, treating apnea first and re-evaluating symptoms and MSLT afterwards help making the diagnosis of narcolepsy. SAS is defined by more than five apnea/hypopnea events per hours of sleep. Persons clinically affected by SAS are frequently sleepy and obese. Otherwise, narcoleptic patients also have an increasing body-mass index than normal subjects, and some, especially children, gain weight after the onset of narcolepsy [4]. This association between narcolepsy and obesity is controversial. Recent studies correlate this link to the reduced serum level of leptin and ghrelin in narcoleptic patients. The suggestive hypothesis is a modulation of these two hormones on Hct system, but, to our knowledge, no studies have been able to find an association between abnormally low serum leptin and Hct deficiency so far [6,39-41]. Thus it can be very hard to differentiate a narcoleptic patient from a SAS-patient, especially in cases of narcolepsy without cataplexy.

IH is a rare condition, defined as a normal or prolonged nocturnal sleep episode that is associated with EDS consisting of prolonged (1-2 hours) sleep episodes of NREM-sleep. Clinically a large majority of members of the task force agreed to separate IH into two entities:

- IH with long sleep time, characterized by EDS, prolonged nocturnal sleep and difficulty in awakening (also called polysymptomatic, or primary, or essential or classic IH)
- IH without long sleep time, remarkable for EDS only (also called monosymptomatic IH, or not otherwise specified hypersomnia, or isolated EDS).

Both of these two entities presented with a reduced mean sleep latency MSLT evaluation and less than two SOREMPs at the MSLT evaluation. Clinically the two conditions are different for the duration of nocturnal sleep. PSG and MSLT test can be questionable for the real evaluation of IH. It can be more useful to perform a 24-h continuous PSG in order to document a major sleep episode at night and daytime sleep episodes, but this procedure is still waiting for standardization and validation. Pathophysiology of IH is almost totally unknown. However a continuum between IH and narcolepsy without cataplexy may be proposed: both the diseases are characterized by normal CSF Hct-1 levels; otherwise, clinically IH without long time sleep stands as isolated EDS, and daytime sleep episodes may be more irresistible and more refreshing than IH with long sleep time, like a narcoleptic attack. This could establish a hypothetical bridge between IH and narcolepsy [33,42-44]. For a systematic update about the diagnosis and the differentiation of narcolepsy and IH see Billiard and coworkers in Sleep Medicine Reviews, 2007 [1].

RH is characterized by recurrent episodes of excessive sleep (at least 16 h/day) lasting from a few days to several weeks. The best defined RH is Kleine-Levine syndrome (KLS), a rare disorder characterized by a constant complaint hypersomnia with cognitive and behavioral disturbances with overeating (in up to 80% of cases) and less frequently hypersexuality during symptomatic episodes. KLS is more frequent in young male patients. Common triggering factors include infections, head trauma, or alcohol abuse. The pathophysiology is totally unknown but many studies suggest a hypothalamic dysfunction. In order to exclude narcolepsy, epilepsy and organic pathology, EEG, PSG-recordings and cerebral imaging are necessary. RH prognosis is unclear, but the evolution is favorable in most cases, with a progressive disappearance of symptoms after 5 years [45,46].

Other sleep disorders, such as chronic sleep deprivation and mood disorders, can produce an EDS caused by the alteration of the normal sleep/wake cycle.

Chronic sleep deprivation syndrome occurs in individuals who fail to obtain for at least 3 months sufficient nocturnal sleep, required to support normally alert wakefulness. Patients report difficulty rising in the morning and sometimes experience sleep drunkenness-like episodes. Patients may also complain of increasing levels of subjective fatigue, mood deterioration, muscular pain, gastrointestinal unrest and visual disturbances. Symptoms usually disappear on weekends and during the holidays. PSG recordings may show a good sleep efficiency (>90%) and a short sleep latency, indicative of a sleep rebound [42,47].

Hypersomnia in *mood disorders* is rarely objective and seems to be more related to the lack of interest and decreased energy inherent to the depressed condition rather than to an increase in sleep or REM-sleep propensity. However, some patient affected by depression can report a hypersomnia similar to that of narcoleptic patients. In that sense hypersomnia can vary from day to day and it is often associated with poor sleep at night. Therefore insomnia and EDS are frequently associated, especially in cases of depression [48]. The association between narcolepsy and depressive mood is frequent whereas several narcoleptic patients develop symptoms of depression. Hypersomnia in narcolepsy can be exacerbated by Depression since the latter can fragmentate normal sleep pattern. This effect is less evident in narcolepsy with cataplexy, where anticataplectic medications are often antidepressant drugs (i.e. Selective Serotonin Reuptake Inhibitors or SSRI and tricyclics) [15,42,49,50].

Frequently narcolepsy overlaps with other REM-sleep disorders, mainly with *REM-sleep Behavior Disorder* (RBD). RBD is a REM-sleep parasomnia characterized by a motor dyscontrol due to the loss of REM-related muscle atonia. Common RBD features are complex, vigorous and frequently violent dream-enacting behavior during REM sleep. This behavior can result in injury to the patient or to the patient's bed partner and has been known to cause fractures, dislocations and even subdural heamatomas. Patients are often male and RBD is often associated with neurodegenerative disorders, especially Parkinson Diseases and Multiple Systemic Atrophy. PSG data can show an increasing thickness in chin EMG tone, called REM Without Atonia (REMWA) [2,51].

The association between narcolepsy and RBD was well-defined in 1992 by Schneck that showed how the 12% of 142 narcoleptic patients had extensive motor dysregulation during REM sleep, and 7% met criteria for RBD [52]. In 1993, a retrospective study analyzed 14 narcoleptic patients, and suggestion was made that sleep motor dyscontrol in narcolepsy may start as a NREM parasomnia in childhood and then "the onset of narcolepsy might represent the turning point for its intrusion into REM sleep" [53]. Therefore it can be speculated narcolepsy and RBD are linked by the same motor dyscontrol during sleep, and often the two entities can overlap. The presence of this altered motor control in this two disease have been recently confirmed by Mattarozzi et al. in 2008 [54]. They studied the clinical, behavioral and PSG correlates of cataplexy in narcoleptic patients discovering as the frequency of cataplectic attack is related to the level of altered motor control during sleep and as this is also modulated by age and gender. The modulation of age and gender in the motor dyscontrol of RBD and narcolepsy has yet been evidenced in a questionnaire study by Nightingale et al. [55]. In their work, they have suggested that all narcoleptic patients, especially those with cataplexy, should be questioned about disturbed sleep and dream-related behavior as they could present RBD-like episodes. Similarly RBD patient should be assessed for symptoms of narcolepsy, particularly if female and of a younger age. To our knowledge, a few cases have reported so far RBD as the first clinical manifestation of a narcolepsy [56].

Narcolepsy is the prototypical example of dissociated sleep/wake phenomena in which components of one state (REM sleep, NREM sleep and wake) appear in another. Our lives are spent in three state of being: wakefulness, REM and NREM. Normally, these states cycle at predictable times and tend to occur independently. Narcolepsy results in an impaired control of these states boundaries. As cataplexy and sleep paralysis represent inappropriate intrusion of REM sleep-related atonia into wakefulness, so RBD episodes can be related to an intrusion of wake behavior into REM sleep [57]. Moreover, iatrogenic RBD episodes can be due to many antidepressants used for cataplexy (i.e. clomipramine and SSRI), which caused REM suppression and increasing REM dream imagery during wakefulness [58,59].

Another feature of altered motor control during sleep in narcoleptics is the presence of a high ratio of *Periodic Limb Movements* (PLM). PLM are characterized by periodic episodes of repetitive and highly stereotypic limb movements during sleep. PLM are frequent in *Restless Legs Syndrome* (RLS). RLS is a sensorimotor disorder characterized by a prototypical complaint of a strong, nearly irresistible urge to move the legs. The onset of symptoms is mainly in the evening, when the subject goes to bed, and they improve with the movement. Approximately 80% of adult RLS and from 63 to 74% of pediatric RLS cases have PLM. The common sleep disturbance in RLS is the difficulty to start sleep, due to the unpleasant sensation related to the legs and to the urgency to move them. The recent etiopathogenetic hypothesis of idiopathic RLS suggests an impairment of the dopaminergic pathway in motor control. The association of PLM during sleep in narcolepsy was first reported in the early 1980 [60]. Several studies have subsequently shown that approximately 50% to 60% of patients with narcolepsy have a PLM index (number of PLM per hour of sleep) of 5 or higher. A recent study has pointed out that narcoleptic patients show a lower PLM periodicity than those affected by RLS. This might be more related to the specific altered microstructure of sleep in narcolepsy rather than the dopaminergic dysfunction typical of RLS [61]. Moreover, PLM were found to be more frequent in HLA DQB1*0602-positive subject with narcolepsy. Hence, the hypocretin deficiency could play a role in the modulation of PLM during sleep in narcoleptic patients [62].

Narcolepsy with cataplexy could be sometimes misdiagnosed as syncope, an epileptic attack, a drop attack or an attack of a histrionic nature, especially when cataplexy is the predominant sign.

Cataplexy is characterized by a sudden drop of muscle tone triggered by emotional factor, especially if positive such as laughter or pleasant surprise rarely by stress, fear, or physical effort [4,63]. All striated muscles can be affected, but cataplectic attack is more often limited to facial muscles or to the arms or legs. Clinical presentation of a cataplectic attack may vary from a simply manifestation of weakness in a part of the body to a real individual collapse with a fall to the ground. It can be noted: facial flickering, jaw tremors, head or jaw dropping, dropping of object, or even episodes of dysarthria. The subject remains entirely conscious during the cataplectic episodes, while deep tendon reflexes are transiently abolished and the H-reflexes are absent. Cataplectic patients can occasionally experience a "status cataplecticus", which comprises continual cataplectic episodes lasting several hours. This state can occur spontaneously but is more often due to an inappropriate withdrawal of anticataplectic/antidepressant drugs [64,65]. A recent case report published by our group showed how the abrupt withdrawal of clomipramine led to a status cataplecticus in a misdiagnosed narcoleptic patient, treated for years as affected by pseudoseizures or recurrent syncope [66]. The loss of the muscle tone in cataplexy rarely concerns suddenly all of muscles of the body. Mostly a cataplectic attack is a slowly and increasing weakness that start from axial muscles (i.e. muscles of neck and proximal muscles of limbs) and then might spread in all part of the body. When all muscles are involved, the patient might experience a fall to the ground that is slowly and graduate.

Syncope is a sudden, transient, spontaneously self-terminating loss of consciousness with complete and prompt recovery. It is mostly due to a metabolic failure of brain or to an insufficient cerebral blood flow. Clinically a syncopal attack can present as a sudden and total weakness of the body, with signs of activated adrenergic system: usually patients can present as sweaty, with a pale-face and cold skin, a low heart-rate and a low or undetectable blood pressure. The onset of syncope may extremely vary from a sensation of diffuse weakness with palpitation, sweat and dizziness (state called presyncope or lipothymia) to a major episode of a sudden and complete loss of consciousness. An accurate cardiac evaluation with a prolonged electrocardiography and an echocardiography can demonstrate an alteration of cardiac rhythm or a valve disorder responsible of the syncopal attack. When a cardiac origin is excluded, an accurate evaluation of the vegetative system can demonstrate an altered blood pressure regulation resulting in hypotension. At the same time a clinical/biochemical evaluation can show a hypoglycemia, that is the main metabolic cause of syncope.

Epileptic seizure is a sudden hypersyncronized discharge of a group of neurons. Clinical manifestation is extremely variable, mainly due to the specific cerebral cortex area involved. Consciousness can be present or not. In narcoleptic patients, especially if children, a cataplectic attack can exist with a narcoleptic one, i.e. the subject can fall to the ground and be asleep. During a cataplectic attack some subjects can experience the possibility to have twitching movements that can be mistaken for the jerking of a seizure [67-69]. Moreover, in the daytime, patient with narcolepsy might show automatic behavior, often manifesting as doing tasks without recall. In these cases, the patient might suddenly say something unfitting or out of context in a conversation, write something inappropriate or illegible, or might drive to a wrong location without memory of the event. Whether automatic behavior is caused by microsleep or cognitive impairment when drowsy it is unknown. It is important to recognize automatic behavior as a symptom of narcolepsy whereas it can be confused with epileptic behavior [4,6]. Thus Narcolepsy was included by Gowers in the so-called "borderland of epilepsy" in 1907. The borderland of epilepsy concerns all of the paroxysmal condition with a clinical manifestation similar to an epileptic seizure and often misdiagnosed with it (syncope, migraine, sleep disorders and vertigo) [70]. For an accurate revision of this concept refer to a recent review by Crompton [71].

Drop attack is a sudden bilateral weakness in antigravitary muscles, often without loss of consciousness. The most important cause of this condition is a transient ischemic attack (TIA) in the posterior areas of the brain, especially in the pons where neural pathways concerning postural tone are localized. In cases of TIA or minor stoke events, some patients might experienced a sudden fall down that could last from few to several minutes, similar to a cataplectic attack. A possible key factor to single out cataplexy from a drop attack is the presence of a positive emotion (i.e. surprise, laughing) triggering the fall.

When narcolepsy started with ancillary features (sleep paralysis or hypnopompic/hypnagogic hallucinations), it can be mistaken as *schizophrenia*. Sleep paralysis and sleep-related hallucinations are considered symptoms of dissociated REM sleep phenomena and not are specific of narcolepsy. Sometimes narcoleptic patients are unable to differentiate these dreams-like episodes from reality, and might occasionally be misdiagnosed as schizophrenics. At the same time, some schizophrenic symptoms can be confounded as narcoleptic ones whereas patients affected by schizophrenia can present as catatonic and unresponsive.

Personality of narcoleptic patients is difficult to assess. The development of a depressive mood in patient with narcolepsy could be due to the interfering of the disease with every aspect of the life. The negative social impact of narcolepsy has been extensively studied and, in particular, it has been highlighted how the disease can impair driving ability, cause car or machine accidents. Narcolepsy also interferes with professional performance leading to unemployement, frequent change in employment, worker's disability or early retirement. In addition to this, narcoleptic patients can develop a histrionic personality that can determine the presence of conversion phenomena. To date, a few cases of young persons affected by "Pseudonarcolepsy" and "Pseudocataplexy" have been reported [72,73]. These terms have been coined to describe a phenomenon, in which a patient presents with the apparent symptoms and signs of narcolepsy, but its origin is psychogenic and they are not really asleep. Etiopathogenesis is still unknown, even if it is likely to be similar to Pseudoseizures or Psychogenic Non Epileptic Seizures (PNES).

PNES are operationally defined as episodes of altered movement, sensation, or experience similar to epilepsy, but caused by a psychological process and not associated with abnormal electrical discharges in the brain. Although physicians as far as back as Hippocrates and Aretaeus differentiated between epileptic and hysterical seizures only the clinical introduction of synchronous video-EEG 30 years ago allowed a definite diagnosis of PNES. Since then our understanding of the semiology of PNES and the clinical context in which they occur has increased rapidly. Despite this, the mean latency between manifestation and diagnosis remains unacceptably long at about 7 years and the three-quarters of patients with PNES are still treated with anticonvulsivants initially [74].

The lifestyle disruption caused by narcolepsy is viewed similar to that caused by epilepsy. Thus, beyond the different and well-defined intrapsychic mechanisms, some cases of these conversion disorders might be interpreted as a social maladjustment, either a maladaptative attempt to get attention, either a case of malingering to keep some benefits (i.e. disability, leave from work, prescription of stimulants) [4]. A correct assessment of the personality and the possible associated psychiatric disorders of narcoleptic patient are important, as many drugs (i.e. benzodiazepine, antidepressant and antipsychotics) can worse the clinical features of narcolepsy, especially the length of EDS.

Conclusion

A correct diagnosis of narcolepsy is very hard especially in childhood when the presence of the four symptoms is not so well-defined. Narcolepsy could be misdiagnosed with many diseases that could mimic its symptoms, especially with the EDS. Cataplexy is the pathognomonic clinical sign that can guide to the correct diagnosis, but sometimes its presence could be confounded with other neurological and psychiatric causes of weakness, loss of normal muscle tone or sudden falls. Diagnosis is clinical but an accurate instrumental evaluation (PSG followed by MLST) is necessary to better assess the alteration of the sleep-wake cycle as well as those of REM phases and of the EDS. This neurophysiological evaluation is mandatory when narcolepsy is not associated with cataplexy or when clinical presentation is not so clear. Narcolepsy has a good outcome, usually improving with specific drugs (modafinil, sodium oxybate, SSRI, tricyclics antidepressant).

Therefore, a misdiagnosis of narcolepsy could lead to an erroneous treatment (i.e. benzodiazepine, antipsychotics and some kind of antidepressants) that can precipitate or exacerbate narcoleptic symptoms worsening quality of life of the patients.

References

[1] Billiard, M. Diagnosis of Narcolepsy and idiopathic hypersomnia. An update based on the International Classification of Sleep Disorders, 2nd edition. *Sleep Medicine Reviews*, 2007, 11, 377-388

[2] American Academy of Sleep Medicine. The International classification of Sleep Disorders: diagnostic and coding manual, 2nd ed. Illinois: AASM, 2005.

[3] Overeem, S; Mignot, E; van Dijk, JG; Lammers, GJ. Narcolepsy: clinical features, new pathophysiologic insights, and future perspectives. *J Clin Neurophysiol.*, 2001 Mar, 18(2), 78-105.

[4] Dauvilliers, Y; Arnulf, I; Mignot, E. Narcolepsy with cataplexy. *Lancet.*, 2007 Feb 10, 369(9560), 499-511. Review

[5] Dauvilliers, Y; Montplaisir, J; Molinari, N; Carlander, B; Ondze, B; Besset, A; Billiard, M. Age at onset of narcolepsy in two large populations of patients in France and Quebec. *Neurology.*, 2001 Dec 11, 57(11), 2029-33

[6] Peterson, PC; Husain, AM. Pediatric narcolepsy. *Brain Dev.*, 2008 Nov, 30(10), 609-23. Epub 2008 Mar 28.

[7] Sakurai, T; Amemiya, A; Ishii, M; Matsuzaki, I; Chemelli, RM; Tanaka, H; Williams, SC; Richarson, JA; Kozlowski, GP; Wilson, S; Arch, JR; Buckingham, RE; Haynes, AC; Carr, SA; Annan, RS; McNulty, DE; Liu, WS; Terrett, JA; Elshourbagy, NA; Bergsma, DJ; Yanagisawa, M. Orexins and orexin receptors: a family of hypothalamic neuropeptides and G protein-coupled receptors that regulate feeding behavior. *Cell.*, 1998 Mar 6, 92(5), 1 page following 696

[8] Sutcliffe, JG; de Lecea, L. The hypocretins: excitatory neuromodulatory peptides for multiple homeostatic systems, including sleep and feeding. *J Neurosci Res.*, 2000 Oct 15, 62(2), 161-8

[9] Krahn, LE; Pankratz, VS; Oliver, L; Boeve, BF; Silber, MH. Hypocretin (orexin) levels in cerebrospinal fluid of patients with narcolepsy: relationship to cataplexy and HLA DQB1*0602 status. *Sleep.*, 2002 Nov 1, 25(7), 733-6

[10] Nishino, S; Okura, M; Mignot, E. Narcolepsy: genetic predisposition and neuropharmacological mechanisms. *Sleep Med Rev.*, 2000 Feb, 4(1), 57-99

[11] Ohayon, MM; Ferini-Strambi, L; Plazzi, G; Smirne, S; Castronovo, V. Frequency of narcolepsy symptoms and other sleep disorders in narcoleptic patients and their first-degree relatives. *J Sleep Res.*, 2005 Dec, 14(4), 437-45

[12] Maret, S; Tafti, M. Genetics of narcolepsy and other major sleep disorders. *Swiss Med Wkly.*, 2005 Nov 19, 135(45-46), 662-5

[13] Dauvilliers, Y; Maret, S; Bassetti, C; Carlander, B; Billiard, M; Touchon, J; Tafti, M. A monozygotic twin pair discordant for narcolepsy and CSF hypocretin-1. *Neurology.*, 2004 Jun 8, 62(11), 2137-8

[14] Smith, AJ; Jackson, MW; Neufing, P; McEvoy, RD; Gordon, TP. A functional autoantibody in narcolepsy. *Lancet.*, 2004 Dec 11-17, 364(9451), 2122-4

[15] Nishino, S. Clinical and neurobiological aspects of narcolepsy. *Sleep Medicine*, 2007, 8, 373-399

[16] Lankford, DA; Wellman, JJ; O'Hara, C. Posttraumatic narcolepsy in mild to moderate closed head injury. *Sleep.*, 1994 Dec, 17(8 Suppl), S25-8

[17] Orellana, C; Villemin, E; Tafti, M; Carlander, B; Besset, A; Billiard, M. Life events in the year preceding the onset of narcolepsy. *Sleep.*, 1994 Dec, 17(8 Suppl), S50-3

[18] Nishino, S; Kanbayashi, T. Symptomatic narcolepsy, cataplexy and hypersomnia, and their implications in the hypothalamic hypocretin/orexin system. *Sleep Med Rev.*, 2005 Aug, 9(4), 269-310. Review

[19] Von Economo, C. Sleep as a problem of localization. *Journal of Nervous and Mental Disorders*, 1930, 71(3), 249-59.

[20] Aldrich, MS; Naylor, MW. Narcolepsy associated with lesions of the diencephalon. *Neurology.*, 1989 Nov, 39(11), 1505-8

[21] Guilleminault, C; Pelayo, R. Narcolepsy in prepubertal children. *Ann Neurol.*, 1998 Jan, 43(1), 135-42

[22] Kryger, MH; Walid, R; Manfreda, J. Diagnoses received by narcolepsy patients in the year prior to diagnosis by a sleep specialist. *Sleep.*, 2002 Feb 1, 25(1), 36-41

[23] Carskadon, MA; Dement, WC; Mitler, MM; Roth, T; Westbrook, PR; Keenan, S. Guidelines for the multiple sleep latency test (MSLT): a standard measure of sleepiness. *Sleep.*, 1986 Dec, 9(4), 519-24

[24] Thorpy, MJ. The clinical use of the Multiple Sleep Latency Test. The Standards of Practice Committee of the American Sleep Disorders Association. *Sleep.*, 1992 Jun, 15(3), 268-76. Review. No abstract available. Erratum in: Sleep 1992 Aug, 15(4), 381

[25] Moscovitch, A; Partinen, M; Guilleminault, C. The positive diagnosis of narcolepsy and narcolepsy's borderland. *Neurology.*, 1993 Jan, 43(1), 55-60

[26] Mitler, MM; Gujavarty, KS; Browman, CP. Maintenance of wakefulness test: a polysomnographic technique for evaluation treatment efficacy in patients with excessive somnolence. *Electroencephalogr Clin Neurophysiol.*, 1982 Jun, 53(6), 658-61

[27] Mitler, MM; Walsleben, J; Sangal, RB; Hirshkowitz, M. Sleep latency on the maintenance of wakefulness test (MWT) for 530 patients with narcolepsy while free of psychoactive drugs. *Electroencephalogr Clin Neurophysiol.*, 1998 Jul, 107(1), 33-8

[28] Juji, T; Satake, M; Honda, Y; Doi, Y. HLA antigens in Japanese patients with narcolepsy. All the patients were DR2 positive. *Tissue Antigens.*, 1984 Nov, 24(5), 316-9

[29] Billiard, M; Seignalet, J. Extraordinary association between HLA-DR2 and narcolepsy. *Lancet.*, 1985 Jan 26, 1(8422), 226-7
[30] Mignot, E. Genetic and Familial aspects of narcolepsy. *Neurology.*, 1998, 50(suppl 1), S16-22.
[31] Kuwata, S; Tokunaga, K; Jin, F; Juji, T; Sasaki, T; Honda, Y. To the Editor: "NARCOLEPSY". *The New England journal of Medicine*, 1991, 270-72.
[32] Nishino, S; Ripley, B; Overeem, S; Lammers, GJ; Mignot, E. Hypocretin (orexin) deficiency in human narcolepsy. *Lancet.*, 2000 Jan 1, 355(9197), 39-40
[33] Mignot, E; Lammers, GJ; Ripley, B; Okun, M; Nevsimalova, S; Overeem, S; Vankova, J; Black, J; Harsh, J; Bassetti, C; Schrader, H; Nishino, S. The role of cerebrospinal fluid hypocretin measurement in the diagnosis of narcolepsy and other hypersomnias. *Arch Neurol.*, 2002 Oct, 59(10), 1553-62
[34] Kanbayashi, T; Inoue, Y; Chiba, S; Aizawa, R; Saito, Y; Tsukamoto, H; Fujii, Y; Nishino, S; Shimizu, T. CSF hypocretin-1 (orexin-A) concentrations in narcolepsy with and without cataplexy and idiopathic hypersomnia. *J Sleep Res.*, 2002 Mar, 11(1), 91-3
[35] Overeem, S; Dalmau, J; Bataller, L; Nishino, S; Mignot, E; Verschuuren, J; Lammers, GJ. Hypocretin-1 CSF levels in anti-Ma2 associated encephalitis. *Neurology.*, 2004 Jan 13, 62(1), 138-40
[36] Nishino, S; Kanbayashi, T; Fujiki, N; Uchino, M; Ripley, B; Watanabe, M; Lammers, GJ; Ishiguro, H; Shoji, S; Nishida, Y; Overeem, S; Toyoshima, I; Yoshida, Y; Shimizu, T; Taheri, S; Mignot, E. CSF hypocretin levels in Guillain-Barré syndrome and other inflammatory neuropathies. *Neurology.*, 2003 Sep 23, 61(6), 823-5.
[37] Baumann, CR; Bassetti, CL. Hypocretins (orexins) and sleep-wake disorders. *Lancet Neurol.*, 2005 Oct, 4(10), 673-82. Review
[38] Malhotra, A; White, DP. Obstructive sleep apnoea. *Lancet.*, 2002 Jul 20, 360(9328), 237-45. Review
[39] Kok, SW; Meinders, AE; Overeem, S; Lammers, GJ; Roelfsema, F; Frölich, M; Pijl, H. Reduction of plasma leptin levels and loss of its circadian rhythmicity in hypocretin (orexin)-deficient narcoleptic humans. *J Clin Endocrinol Metab.*, 2002 Feb, 87(2), 805-9
[40] Sakurai, T. Roles of orexins and orexin receptors in central regulation of feeding behavior and energy homeostasis. *CNS Neurol Disord Drug Targets.*, 2006 Jun, 5(3), 313-25. Review

[41] Arnulf, I; Lin, L; Zhang, J; Russell, IJ; Ripley, B; Einen, M; Nevsimalova, S; Bassetti, C; Bourgin, P; Nishino, S; Mignot, E. CSF versus serum leptin in narcolepsy: is there an effect of hypocretin deficiency? *Sleep.*, 2006 Aug 1, 29(8), 1017-24

[42] Dauvilliers, Y. Differential diagnosis in hypersomnia. *Curr Neurol Neurosci Rep.*, 2006 Mar, 6(2), 156-62. Review

[43] Billiard, M; Dauvilliers, Y. Idiopathic Hypersomnia. *Sleep Med Rev.*, 2001 Oct, 5(5), 349-358

[44] Dauvilliers, Y; Baumann, CR; Carlander, B; Bischof, M; Blatter, T; Lecendreux, M; Maly, F; Besset, A; Touchon, J; Billiard, M; Tafti, M; Bassetti, CL. CSF hypocretin-1 levels in narcolepsy, Kleine-Levin syndrome, and other hypersomnias and neurological conditions. *J Neurol Neurosurg Psychiatry.*, 2003 Dec, 74(12), 1667-73.

[45] Critchley, M. Periodic hypersomnia and megaphagia in adolescent males. *Brain.*, 1962 Dec, 85, 627-56.

[46] Arnulf, I; Zeitzer, JM; File, J; Farber, N; Mignot, E. Kleine-Levin syndrome: a systematic review of 186 cases in the literature. *Brain.*, 2005 Dec, 128(Pt 12), 2763-76. Epub 2005 Oct 17. Review

[47] Carskadon, MA; Dement, WC. Cumulative effects of sleep restriction on daytime sleepiness. *Psychophysiology*, 1981 Mar, 18(2), 107-13

[48] Billiard, M; Dolenc, L; Aldaz, C; Ondze, B; Besset, A. Hypersomnia associated with mood disorders: a new perspective. *J Psychosom Res.*, 1994, 38 Suppl 1, 41-7

[49] Broughton, R; Ghanem, Q; Hishikawa, Y; Sugita, Y; Nevsimalova, S; Roth, B. Life effects of narcolepsy in 180 patients from North America, Asia and Europe compared to matched controls. *Can J Neurol Sci.*, 1981 Nov, 8(4), 299-304

[50] Roth, B; Nevsimalova, S. Depresssion in narcolepsy and hypersommia. *Schweiz Arch Neurol Neurochir Psychiatr.*, 1975, 116(2), 291-300

[51] Schenck, CH; Bundlie, SR; Ettinger, MG; Mahowald, MW. Chronic behavioral disorders of human REM sleep: a new category of parasomnia. *Sleep.*, 1986 Jun, 9(2), 293-308

[52] Schenck, CH; Mahowald, MW. Motor dyscontrol in narcolepsy: rapid-eye-movement (REM) sleep without atonia and REM sleep behavior disorder. *Ann Neurol.*, 1992 Jul, 32(1), 3-10

[53] Mayer, G; Meier-Ewert, K. Motor dyscontrol in sleep of narcoleptic patients (a lifelong development?). *J Sleep Res.*, 1993 Sep, 2(3), 143-148

[54] Mattarozzi, K; Bellucci, C; Campi, C; Cipolli, C; Ferri, R; Franceschini, C; Mazzetti, M; Russo, PM; Vandi, S; Vignatelli, L; Plazzi, G. Clinical, behavioural and polysomnographic correlates of cataplexy in patients with narcolepsy/cataplexy. *Sleep Med.*, 2008 May, 9(4), 425-33. Epub 2007 Aug 2

[55] Nightingale, S; Orgill, JC; Ebrahim, IO; de Lacy, SF; Agrawal, S; Williams, A. The association between narcolepsy and REM behavior disorder (RBD). *J. Sleep Med.*, 2005 May, 6(3), 253-8.

[56] Bonakis, A; Howard, RS; Williams, A. Narcolepsy presenting as REM sleep behaviour disorder. *Clin Neurol Neurosurg.*, 2008 May, 110(5), 518-20. Epub 2008 Mar 17

[57] Mahowald, MW; Schenck, CH. Status dissociatus--a perspective on states of being. *Sleep.*, 1991 Feb, 14(1), 69-79. Review

[58] Attarian, HP; Schenck, CH; Mahowald, MW. Presumed REM sleep behavior disorder arising from cataplexy and wakeful dreaming. *Sleep Med.*, 2000 Apr 1, 1(2), 131-133.

[59] Bental, E; Lavie, P; Sharf, B. Severe hypermotility during sleep in treatment of cataplexy with clomipramine. *Isr J Med Sci.*, 1979 Jul, 15(7), 607-9

[60] Coleman, RM; Pollak, CP; Weitzman, ED. Periodic movements in sleep (nocturnal myoclonus): relation to sleep disorders. *Ann Neurol.*, 1980 Oct, 8(4), 416-21

[61] Ferri, R; Zucconi, M; Manconi, M; Bruni, O; Ferini-Strambi, L; Vandi, S; Montagna, P; Mignot, E; Plazzi, G. Different periodicity and time structure of leg movements during sleep in narcolepsy/cataplexy and restless legs syndrome. *Sleep.*, 2006 Dec 1, 29(12), 1587-94

[62] Hong, SC; Hayduk, R; Lim, J; Mignot, E. Clinical and polysomnographic features in DQB1*0602 positive and negative narcolepsy patients: results from the modafinil clinical trial. *Sleep Med.*, 2000 Feb 1, 1(1), 33-39

[63] Thorpy, MJ. Cataplexy associated with narcolepsy: epidemiology, pathophysiology and management. *CNS Drugs*, 2006, 20(1), 43-50. Review

[64] Overeem, S; Reijntjes, R; Huyser, W; Lammers, GJ; van Dijk, JG. Corticospinal excitability during laughter: implications for cataplexy and the comparison with REM sleep atonia. *J Sleep Res.*, 2004 Sep, 13(3), 257-64.

[65] Poryazova, R; Siccoli, M; Werth, E; Bassetti, CL. Unusually prolonged rebound cataplexy after withdrawal of fluoxetine. *Neurology.*, 2005 Sep 27, 65(6), 967-8

[66] Calabrò, RS; Savica, R; Laganà, A; Magaudda, A; Imbesi, D; Gallitto, G; La Spina, P; Musolino, R. Status cataplecticus misdiagnosed as recurrent syncope. *Neurol Sci.*, 2007 Dec, 28(6), 336-8. Epub 2008 Jan 4.

[67] Zeman, A; Douglas, N; Aylward, R. Lesson of the week: Narcolepsy mistaken for epilepsy. *BMJ.*, 2001 Jan 27, 322(7280), 216-8.

[68] Robinson, A; Guilleminault, C. Narcolepsy. In: S. Chokroverty (Ed.), *Sleep disorders medicine*. Boston: Butterworth Heinemann, 1999.

[69] Macleod, S; Ferrie, C; Zuberi, SM. Symptoms of narcolepsy in children misinterpreted as epilepsy. *Epileptic Disord.*, 2005 Mar, 7(1), 13-7

[70] Gowers, WR. The Border-land of Epilepsy: Faints, Vagal Attacks, Vertigo, Migraine and Sleep Symptoms and Their treatment. London: Churchill, 1907.

[71] Crompton, DE; Berkovic, SF. The borderland of epilepsy: clinical and molecular features of phenomena that mimic epileptic seizures. *Lancet Neurol.*, 2009 Apr, 8(4), 370-81. Review

[72] Hvidsten, S; Bates, G. Pseudonarcolepsy in an 11-year-old boy. *Clin Child Psychol Psychiatry.*, 2008 Oct, 13(4), 585-91. Review

[73] Krahn, LE; Hansen, MR; Shepard, JW. Pseudocataplexy. *Psychosomatics.*, 2001 Jul-Aug, 42(4), 356-8.

[74] Reuber, M; Elger, CE. Psychogenic nonepileptic seizures: review and update. *Epilepsy Bhav.*, 2003 Jun, 4(3), 205-16. Review.

In: Nacrolepsy: Symptoms, Causes...
Editors: G. Santos et al. pp. 87-106
ISBN: 978-1-60876-645-1

Chapter IV

Narcolepsy in Children

Sona Nevsimalova*
Department of Neurology, Charles University, 1st Faculty of Medicine and Teaching Hospital, Prague, Czech Republic

Abstract

Childhood narcolepsy can be a key to our understanding of the pathogenesis of this disease. The most recent research has been focused on the possibility of autoimmune-mediated destruction of hypocretin/orexin-containing neurons particularly in children and adolescents, and on early diagnosis. However, the diagnosis of childhood narcolepsy is more difficult than in later life, particularly for the specific symptoms appearing in early childhood. Daytime sleepiness has a longer duration in toddlers and preschool children and cataplectic attacks are often mistaken for astatic-myoclonic epileptic seizures. Young patients seem less disturbed by cataplexy than adults; lacking self-awareness, they continue to watch cartoons, conduct other activities or joke even in the presence of multiple repetitive attacks. A semipermanent state of facial muscle weakness with occasional exacerbations is a marked feature there. Toddlers and preschool children are unable to express states of hypnagogic/hypnopompic hallucinations and/or sleep paralysis in their own words, hence, clinical

* Corresponding author: Department of Neurology, Charles University, 1st Faculty of Medicine and Teaching Hospital, Katerinska 30, 128 00 Prague 2, Czech Republic, Telephone: +420-224965562, Mobile +420-607810139, Fax: +420-224922678, E-mail: snevsi@LF1.cuni.cz

evaluation of narcolepsy is particularly critical as normative data for MSLT corresponding to different children's age are not available. Attention should, therefore, be paid to sleep diary, pediatric sleepiness scale, actigraphy, long-term polysomnographic monitoring, human leukocyte tests and hypocretin evaluation. Complementary methods including neuroimaging and genetic tests are necessary to exclude secondary (symptomatic) cases, particularly if cataplectic attacks predominate. The treatment and management of pediatric cases require a specific approach. These reasons contributed to the development of the international PHEA (Physical Health Executive Agency) project devoted to rare pediatric neurological diseases (nEUroped) covering also childhood narcolepsy. Ten European countries participate in this research centered mainly on patient-related optimization of medical care (diagnosis and therapy), on interaction and collaboration between centers, patients and their family members, and on recommendations for young narcoleptics´ psychological and social needs.

Introduction

Retrospective studies suggest that about half of adults with narcolepsy had onset of symptoms since the youth [1], but a large prospective series identified only 5% of the cases as prepubertal [2]. The estimation of diagnosis in adults is all too often delayed more than 10 years [3], and many cases stay under-diagnosed. In children the complaint is diagnosed earlier; according to some Sleep Centers within two years of the disease onset [4, 5]. The prevalence of narcolepsy-cataplexy ranges from 0.025 to 0.40 % [6, 7, 8], unfortunately, data on the incidence and prevalence for narcolepsy in children are missing. One of the most important reviews of pediatric cases presented by Challamel et al. [9], drawing upon literatury sources and her own series of 97 children. She found their mean age at onset to be 9 years with 8 % aged 5 years or less.

According to some authors [6, 10] the age at onset can differentiate patients with a positive family history of narcolepsy with an earlier onset from those without a family history, in whom the disease manifests itself later in life. Clinical and polygraphic findings may indicate that young age at onset is associated with increased severity of the condition, with a higher frequency of cataplexy and decreased mean sleep latency on the Multiple Sleep Latency Test (MSLT). However, our recent findings [11] do not confirm the presumption that clinical severity depends on the age at onset. On a cohort of 105 patients, we found no relation between the number of sleep and cataplectic attacks and the age at onset, nor did subjective Epworth Sleepiness Score (ESS) show any significant dependence. However, earlier onset of the disease correlated with shorter MSLT mean latency. Further longitudinal follow-up of cases with childhood and adulthood onset is desirable to draw a conclusion focused on the prognosis of childhood cases.

Pathogenesis of the Disease and Childhood Cases

An autoimmune-mediated destruction of hypocretin (Hcrt)/orexin containing neurons has been suggested for more than 5 years [12]. The body's immune system was believed to play a role in killing Hcrt-making cells, primarily because of literary data showing a link between narcolepsy and a variant for the human leukocyte antigen. According to recent study, HLA DQA1*0102 and DQB1*0602 are primarily susceptibility factors for narcolepsy [13].

Some studies [14, 15, 16] are focused on early detection of the disease and on the chances for efficacious autoimmune suppressive treatment using intravenous immunoglobulins (IVIGs). However, these were open labeled trials, all positive effects were reported only subjectively with respect to a possible placebo effect. Other authors did not confirm this experience as regards steroid treatment [17]. Therefore, there is a strong need for randomized, double blind placebo-controlled trials with IVIGs at the very early onset of the disease in children and adolescents to verify the effect of autoimmune suppressive treatment.

An exciting whole-genome scans study allowing the analysis of thousands of genetic variation of 1.800 people carrying the same HLA gene variant (800 suffering from narcolepsy-cataplexy) was recently published by Mignot´s group [18]. Procedures devised by the Genome Wide Association (GWA) in Causians with replication in three ethnic groups, they found a highly significant correlation with polymorphisms in the T-cell receptor alpha (TCRA) locus. This is the first documented genetic involvement of the TCRA locus, the major receptor for HLA-peptide presentation, in any disease. Narcolepsy thus will provide new insights into how HLA-TCR interaction contributes to organ specific autoimmune targeting. It is highly probable that HLA and this T cell variant interact in a way that kills Hcrt cells. How exactly this interaction is triggered is a theme to be solved in future studies.

Although susceptibility to narcolepsy, like many autoimmune conditions, is largely genetically determined, environmental factors can have a launching role as triggers for the disease manifestation. From this point of view, pediatric cases can have a key role in the pathophysiology of the disease, and, indeed, a great effort is currently being exerted to deal with this problem. One of the most recent study shows that streptococcal infections can be probably a significant environmental trigger for narcolepsy [19].

Childhood Narcolepsy - Specific Clinical Features

The clinical diagnosis of childhood narcolepsy can be more difficult than in later life, particularly for the specific clinical features appearing in early childhood compared with adults.

1. Excessive Daytime Sleepiness

Excessive daytime sleepiness is usually the first symptom of narcolepsy, a complaint present in all patients regardless of age [20]. However, overwhelming sleep attacks in children are constant and, as a rule, of longer duration than in adults. In some patients chronic waxing and waning of drowsiness during the day with periodic superimposed sleep episodes can be observed. The children are sleepy during lessons at school, on return at home in the afternoon their naps can last up to 2-3 hours without being restorative [21, 22, 23]. Sometimes, confusional arousals with features of sleep drunkenness may be present [4, 24]. Owing to inattentiveness due to permanent sleepiness they have school problems including poor progress and impaired social integration. Due to prolonged sleep attack, they have less time for play or for homework. In young children, restlessness and motor hyperactivity can sometimes overcome the drowsiness [25] and gived rise to behavioral problems.

In many childhood cases, excessive daytime sleepiness is not immediately recognized as abnormal before cataplexy appears [2].

2. Cataplexy

Cataplectic attacks provoked by strong emotion (most often by laughter), reported in 80.5% of all idiopathic cases [9], are as common in children as in adults. However, on a video-analysis of children´s cataplectic attacks [24] illustrated in some patients a clear rostro-caudal progression of the muscle weakness arising in the facial district and then spreading to the trunk, arms, and lower limbs, and finally leading to a fall. In a third of the observed cases, Serra et al. [24] found a typical feature of "cataplectic facies" with repetitive mouth opening, tongue protrusion and drooping eyelids appearing close to disease onset (Figure 1). This semipermanent state of facial muscle weakness with occasional exacerbations precedes typical cataplexy triggered by emotion and could been mistaken for sleepiness. The duration of a single cataplectic spells could last only one or two seconds. Young patients seem less disturbed by cataplexy than adults; due to a lack of self-awareness during such attacks, they will go on watching cartoons, conducting other activities or joking even in the presence of multiple repetitive attacks.

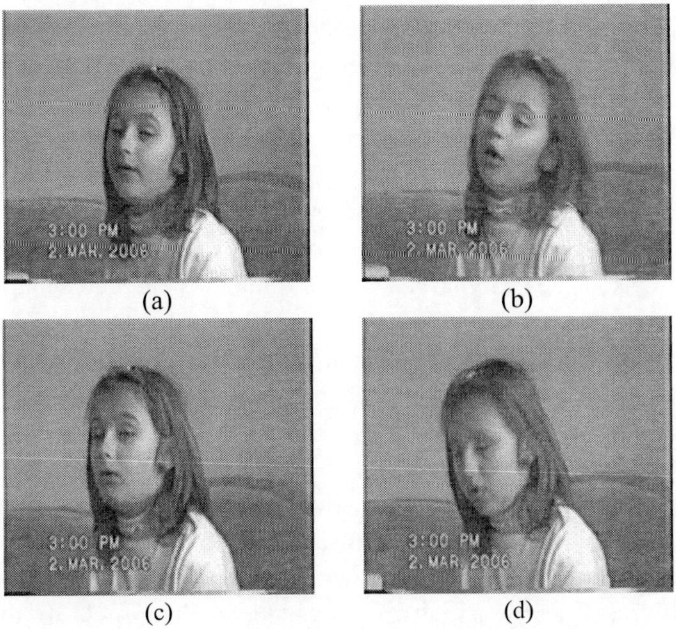

Figure 1. A typical feature of "cataplectic facies" during a short cataplectic attacks appearing close to disease onset in an 8 year-old girl.

However, cataplexy need not be present during the initial years of the disease and/or if it is present, it may, at first, be only sporadic. The children tend to attach little significance to such attack. Sometimes they may feel ashamed, which is when repeated, target-oriented questioning is needed to obtain the required anamnestic data. In rare cases, an isolated appearance of cataplexy preceding excessive daytime sleepiness may pose a diagnostic problem and can be misdiagnosed as astatic-myoclonic epileptic seizures [26, 27].

3. Additional REM Sleep Symptoms and Nocturnal Sleep Disturbances

The presence of **hypnagogic/hypnopompic** hallucinations varied in children from 39 % in the multicentric series [9] up to more than 50 % in others [25, 24, 20]. Contrary to adults, in whom the hallucinations are usually frightening, in children they may have simple forms (colored circles, images of animals or people). Rarely, if there is an emotional content, they can be confused with sleep terrors, nightmares, or panic attacks, in adolescents even with schizophrenia. Unlike schizophrenia, in which the verbal-auditory sensory mode predominates and which appears also without connection to sleep, in narcoleptic patients multisensoric hallucinations are exclusively bound to falling asleep and/or awakening [28, 29]. Hallucinations are often so realistic that patients may believe that they are real [20]. Their occurrence is frequently associated with **sleep paralysis** [27]. Sleep paralysis with inability to move occurs due to persisting REM atonia after awakening while respiratory and extraocular movements are preserved. The episodes usually lasts seconds to minutes and end spontaneously. They can be interrupted if the affected child is touched, shaken or spoken by his/her parents [30]. Sleep paralysis accompanies childhood narcolepsy a little less frequently [9, 25, 24, 20] than hypnagogic/ hypnopompic hallucination (in 29-60 %).

Toddlers and early preschool children are not able to describe states of hypnagogic/hypnopompic hallucinations and/or sleep paralysis in their own words so that clinical evaluation is difficult. The bizarre nature of hallucinations and sleep paralysis may confuse children who are then too embarrassed to discuss their problems; consequently, parents must sometimes help to clarify the child´s experience [23].

Disrupted nocturnal sleep is a frequent complaint of adult patients, but usually it is not reported spontaneously by the parents of affected children. If targeted questions are used, up to 89 % answers are positive [24]. The inability to maintain sleep at night coupled with excessive sleepiness during the day can be very frustrating to patients and family members alike. It can lead to poor sleep habits with children often doing homework at odd hours of the night [20]. Nocturnal sleep disturbances appearing with vivid dreams and often with nightmares could be misdiagnosed as parasomnias. On the other hand, REM behavior may appear even as one of the first symptoms of the disease [31]. Recently, Cyrille and Arnulf [32] brought out the fact that nearly 20 % of narcoleptic patients can sleep long during the night. According to our experience, this subgroup of patients comes particularly from among young patients.

Unlike adults, children suffering from narcolepsy often report **sleep drunkenness** (confusional arousals, sleep inertia) after morning awakening lasting 15-30 minutes. Parents may experience major conflicts with the child because of confusional arousals, particularly when the children are woken-up in the early morning for school [25]. Similarly as morning sleep inertia, also **automatic behavior** during the day can imitate in children states of cloaked consciousness of epileptic origin and can be misinterpreted for partial seizure epilepsy.

4. Further Specific Features of Childhood Narcolepsy

Children and adolescents with narcolepsy often present **personality and behavioral changes.** They become more introverted, and are prone to feelings of inferiority, sorrowfulness, emotional lability or sometimes irritability or even aggressiveness. They also show significantly higher rates of behavioral problems and depression [30]. Interpersonal conflicts are easy to arise within the family and at school [33]. Poor attention and concentration, and disciplinary problems due to sleepiness in class lead to false accusations of drug use. The quality of life in comparison with controls is poorer. Their worse scores of the diseases severity correlate with many aspects of behavior, emotional state, quality of life, educational progress and impact on the children´s families [30].

Obesity as another frequent co-existing problem in childhood narcolepsy (sometimes accompanied by nocturnal eating disorder) may occur in at least 1/4 of narcoleptic children [34, 25]. The tendency towards increased weight gain is manifested relatively early in the course of the disorder [35] and occurs despite of lower caloric intake and does not appear to be due to inactivity or medication causing weight gain [36, 37, 38, 39]. The mechanism of weight gain is thought to be related to abnormal Hcrt and leptin levels and impaired energy metabolism [40, 37, 41, 42]. However, recently published detailed study [43] stopped short of supporting leptin as a mediator of body mass index (BMI) increase in narcolepsy, and another study devoted to eating disorder and metabolism in narcoleptic patients [44] revealed that narcoleptics have a lower basal metabolism than controls. Although they eat less than healthy subjects, they have tendency to being overweight. Both lower metabolism and subtle changes in eating behavior (rather than in calorie intake) are responsible for the positive energy balance leading to increased BMI in adults and probably in narcoleptic children as well.

Severe narcolepsy-cataplexy cases in children rarely arise in close temporal association with obesity and primary **precocious puberty** [45]. This association reflects probably a broadly based hypothalamic abnormality.

In what is another particular feature of childhood, there is a high frequency of **secondary (symptomatic) narcolepsy-cataplexy cases** involving 1/5 – 1/3 of all paediatric patients [9, 21]. Most frequently they are caused by structural brain lesion. In comparison with idiopathic cases, the age at onset in symptomatic ones is lower (6 years on average) with cataplexy as the predominant symptom. Up to 1/4 of the patients described in the relevant literature [9] have a history of status cataplecticus. The most extensive study of secondary cases was published by Nishino and Kanbayashi [46]. They summarized 26 cases of secondary childhood narcolepsy-cataplexy, 15 of them with isolated symptomatic cataplexy or cataplexy-like attacks. The most frequent causes were inherited diseases and brain tumors. While symptomatic cataplexy was frequently associated with non-hypothalamic structures, and the most frequent causes were inherited diseases (Coffin-Lowry syndrome, Norrie disease and Niemann-Pick disease), in symptomatic narcolepsy-cataplexy the hypothalamic region was affected as a rule. The most frequent structural abnormalities included brain tumors particularly in the suprasellar region, predominantly craniopharyngeomas [47] with Niemann-Pick disease type C prevailing among genetic diseases [48, 49] followed by the Prader-Willi syndrome, more rarely by some other structural hypothalamic lesions caused by cerebral palsy, multiple sclerosis and/or some less well-known neurological abnormalities [9].

Therefore, careful history taking with neurological examination and neuroimaging methods (computerized tomography, CT or, better still, magnetic resonance imaging, MRI) should clarify the secondary etiology of the disease and, in specific cases should be coupled with genetic examination.

Diagnostic Evaluation

The diagnostic symptoms of narcolepsy are usually less typical in young children. Daytime sleepiness may be difficult to recognize in early childhood, children can be misidentified as hyperactive, in the older ones as learning disabled, inattentive and lazy. Cataplexy in young age may be missed, disregarded as clumsiness or misdiagnosed as epileptic drop attacks. Moreover, young children are unable to explain their feelings during sleep paralysis and/or hypnagogic hallucinations [27]. Diagnostic criteria for toddlers and preschool children based on sleep studies are missing and so is the pathological limit of mean latency of MSLT for early school children.

The **sleep diary** illustrating the amount of daytime and nocturnal sleep is a useful method for young children. It should rule out sleep-wake cycle irregularity caused by the wrong kind of regime and poor sleep hygiene. Sleep log can be completed in younger children by their parents, in older children by themselves. False excessive daytime sleepiness linked to the delayed (or advanced) sleep phase syndrome can also be eliminated by actigraphic recordings. **Actigraphy** seems to be a useful screening method even in cases of childhood narcolepsy to illustrate repeated naps [4, 21]. Owing to a longer duration of sleep attacks, this method is better applicable in young children than in older ones and adults (Figure 2).

In toddlers and young preschool children, continuous **24h lasting ambulatory polygraphic monitoring** can serve as a useful diagnostic method and can supply useful information also in older children [50]. It can confirm daytime sleep onset REM periods (SOREMs) accompanied by sleep attacks as well as detect cataplectic attacks (Figure 3).

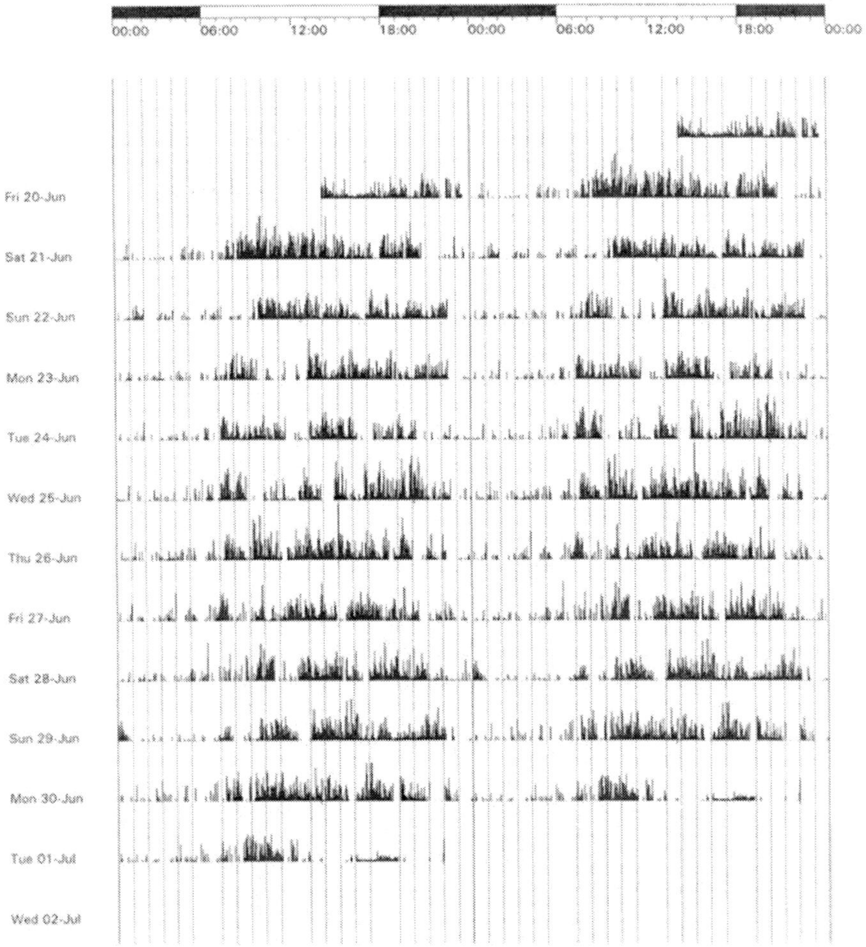

Figure 2. Actigraphic record of a 14-year old girl with narcolepsy-cataplexy. Note the presence of repeated periods of decreased movement activity marking her daily naps.

In children over 6 years of age [24] **overnight polysomnography** (PSG) in conjunction with daytime MSLT is usually used. Nocturnal PSG eliminates other causes of excessive daytime sleepiness such as sleep disordered breathing and/or periodic limb movements. However, their presence does not rule out the presence of narcolepsy, they can coexist in a significant minority of narcoleptic patients [51]. Overnight polygraphic sleep records also exclude parasomnias as a cause of fragmented and unquiet nocturnal sleep and/or verified REM behavior disorder as one of the possible symptoms of narcolepsy [31].

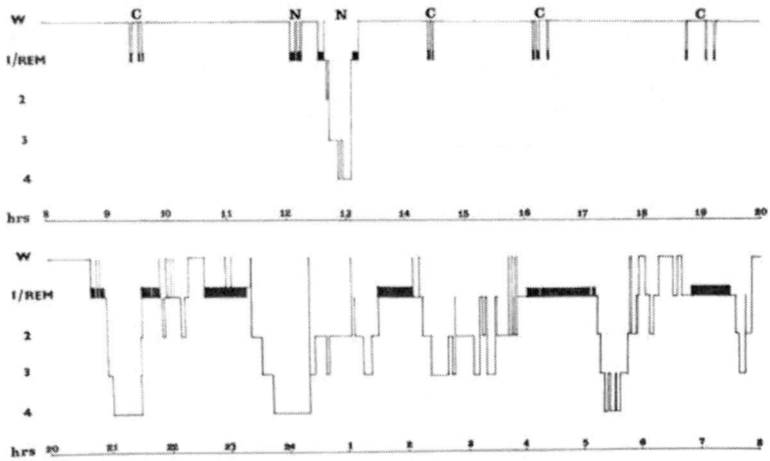

Figure 3. Polygraphic monitoring lasting 24h in a 3-year old child with narcolepsy-cataplexy. Listening to a funny story, read out by his mother, evoked cataplectic attacks.

Multiple sleep latency test (MSLT) is used as a standard diagnostic method [52] in school children, however the exact pathological limit for mean sleep latency is not known. Particularly adolescents may develop physiological hypersomnia [53]. In preadolescents, a mean sleep latency of less than 10 minutes can be assumed as abnormal [21]. In some situations, children may become hypervigilant during the MSLT with marked alerting to minor stimuli, and the test can be invalidated by technical problems. Generally speaking, MSLT in children requires much more patience from technicians, and may sometimes need also a number of repeats [25, 54].

In children as well as in adults, two or more episodes of SOREM are considered pathological. Many authors describe the highest amount of SOREMs just at the onset of the disease [2, 10, 11]. However, Einen and coauthors [5] collected a group of 51 children with the onset both before and after puberty. They found a significantly higher MSLT latency (4.3±1.3 min) in pre-pubertal children than in post-pubertal (1.3±0.3) patients with a similar mean of SOREMs.

This finding is in accordance with our experience. Even in some early-stage cases the polygraphic criteria may not have been met. The latency between clinical symptoms of narcolepsy and the presence of SOREMs in MSLT can last months [55], or even longer, particularly in cases with a delayed development of cataplexy.

Human leukocyte antigen typing is a useful diagnostic tool particularly in children because of its non-invasiveness. The presence of the DQB1*0602 haplotype adds a great deal to the diagnostic probability of narcolepsy, though DQB1*0602 negativity does not exclude it. Particularly, in children with multiple-case history in families, where the age of the disease onset used to be younger, negative HLA findings have no informative value [56, 57]. The absence of DQB1*0602 in young children with sporadic narcolepsy may also indicate a symptomatic origin of the disease. HLA examination has a predictive value in children with excessive daytime sleepiness, though currently free from cataplectic attacks [21].

Cerebrospinal fluid (CSF) **hypocretin-1** (Hcrt-1) **evaluation** is a very valuable diagnostic marker in children, especially where the Hcrt-1 level is undetectable. However, diagnostic lumbar puncture is an invasive method and some parents do not accept it in their child. In prepubertal children undetectable Hcrt-1 levels in CSF appear together with the first clinical manifestations of narcolepsy-cataplexy [55], even before polysomnographic criteria are met. The declining level of CSF Hcrt-1 is closely related predominantly to HLA positive cases [58]. The situation is even more complicated in HLA-negative narcolepsy-cataplexy cases and/or in narcolepsy without cataplexy where the CSF Hcrt-1 level is usually normal. An undetectable Hcrt-1 level can be one of the factors predicting a later appearance of cataplexy, especially in children so far diagnosed only with isolated excessive daytime sleepiness.

Treatment and Management of Pediatric Cases

According to generally accepted opinion [2, 25, 21, 20] there is no specific treatment for narcolepsy in children as distinct from adults as both nonpharmacological and pharmacological means are applied. Children and their parents should be informed about the lifelong nature of the disease and about the need for long-term treatment. It is important to start the treatment in school age as early as possible to avoid problems of poor achievement. Nevertheless, any drug therapy must take into account possible adverse effects. The treatment thus balances avoidance of adverse effects, including tolerance, with the need to maintain an active life. Stimulant (and incidentally anticataplectic) medication represents only one component of the therapeutic program.

The most effective **non-pharmacological** treatment for daytime sleepiness is based on regular sleep-wake schedules and planned naps. At least two planned daytime naps at lunchtime and during the afternoon (between 4 and 5) are recommended in pre-pubertal and pubertal children to enhance refreshment, daytime alertness and performance [59].

Children should be encouraged to participate in after-school and sports activities; similarly, a well-designed exercise program can have a stimulating effect. Adolescents should be counseled not to drive, use alcohol or engage in dangerous activities while drowsy. Close cooperation between teachers in school and parents is desirable. Monitoring for emotional problems and depression, and providing appropriate career counseling are also important.

Pharmacological therapy is mainly focused on lowering the amount of daytime sleepiness and rate of cataplectic attacks, if they are frequent and annoy the child. *Methylphenidate* is one of the older stimulants used for decades for daytime sleepiness curtailment and sometimes also for reducing cataplexy attacks. Though there are no studies evaluating the effect of methylphenidate in children suffering from narcolepsy, the drug has been used in other pediatric conditions such as attention deficit hyperactivity disorder (ADHD), indeed, some directions for dosage in children are available [60, 20]. The initial dose is 5 mg in the morning with upward titration by 5-10 mg/day at weekly intervals. In children weighting less than 25 kg, the methylphenidate dose should not exceed 45 mg/day, usually divided in morning and midday applications. Beside immediate-release formulation (e.g. Ritalin), also extended release preparations (e.g. Concerta) with a biphasic peak lasting all day are available. As a method of choice, methylphenidate as a patch is in use (Daytrana). In either case, the morning dosage and/or morning patch application will guarantee a long lasting effect for the whole day *Amphetamine and dextroamphetamine* are less used stimulants in pediatric practice. According to extremely rare experience from the youngest children [61, 56, 57], any treatment with stimulants should be postponed until preschool age. In toddlers, the metabolic pathways involved in the processing of stimulants may not yet be fully matured.

The most common medication used for children against daytime sleepiness is *modafinil* [62, 20, 23], however, no extensive pharmacological studies are available for the use of modafinil in children with narcolepsy. Ivanenko et al. [62] recommend doses comparable to those in adults (200-400 mg/day). More detailed therapeutic studies are available in children suffering from ADHD [63]. The initial dosage varies according to age between 100-200 mg/day in the morning.

Modafinil can be co-administred in children with other stimulants to enhance the alerting effect of either drug alone.

If cataplexy is the dominant symptom, antidepressants such as *clomipramine* (tricyclic antidepressant), *venlafaxin* (serotonin and norepinephrine reuptake inhibitor, SSRI), and/or *fluoxetine* (SSRI) are usually prescribed. The recommended dosage should be based on body weight, and the initial dose should be of the lowest potency and highest efficacy [23].

Sodium oxybate is the first choice drug for treatment of cataplexy in adults. However, data for children are scarce. One study with 8 children [64] did show a reduction of cataplexy in this age group as well. With the doses ranging from 3 to 7 g/night, the drug was relatively well tolerated particularly by adolescent narcoleptics and found as efficacious there as in adults. Sodium oxybate improves cataplexy, daytime sleepiness as well as fragmented nocturnal sleep. It seems to be an efficacious drug in the treatment of serious cases of childhood narcolepsy-cataplexy. However, more experience of randomized, double blind placebo-controlled trials is still needed in children, which is why in many countries sodium oxybate has so far been reserved for post-pubertal children.

An *autoimmune suppressive course of treatment* (intravenously supplemented immunoglobulins) in the earliest stages of the disease is believed to be one of the most effective possibilities [14, 15, 16], albeit in need of more clarification. On the other hand, there is no benefit in orally administered steroid treatment [17], or in plasmapheresis [65]. The effect of autoimmune suppressive treatment is still unclear so that further studies aimed at immunomodulation are needed.

Conclusion

The diagnosis of narcolepsy in childhood is difficult and pediatricians should include narcolepsy in their differential diagnosis. A clinical examination covering detailed anamnestic data and following auxiliary examinations is useful for diagnosis. Increased daytime somnolence may sometimes be the only sign for a number of years; the sleep attacks become increasingly long, lasting up to hours; confusional arousals with features of sleep drunkenness may be present. Cataplexy may develop with delay, and in addition, some children are too embarrassed to discuss their symptoms. The narcoleptic tetrad is only exceptionally present. In some cases polygraphic criteria may be missing in the early stage of the disease. However, looking for the HLA-DQB1*0602 haplotype and undetectable CSF Hcrt-1 levels will greatly facilitate diagnosis. Beside the typical symptoms, some additional features including obesity and nocturnal bulimia may appear. Also poor school performance and emotional disorder are common complaints. At all events neuroimaging examination, if necessary, genetic tests should be used to exclude any secondary etiology of the disease. Treatment should start as early as possible to avoid the development of problems with progress at school, and close parent-teacher cooperation should be maintained. In any case, treatment and management of pediatric cases require a specific approach.

These reasons contributed to the development of the international European PHEA (Physical Health Executive Agency) project devoted to rare pediatric neurological diseases (nEUroped) including also childhood narcolepsy. Ten European countries participate in this research focusing mainly on optimized medical care for the patients (diagnosis and therapy), on interaction and collaboration between centers, patients and their family members, and on recommendations for psychological and social needs of young narcoleptics.

Acknowledgment

Supported by the Czech Ministry of Education and Youth grant No 0021620849 and by PHEA project nEUroped.

References

[1] McKenna, C; McNicholas, F. Childhood onset narcolepsy. A case report. *European Child and Adolescent Psychiatry*, 2003, 12, 43-47.

[2] Guilleminault, C; Pelayo, R. Narcolepsy in prepubertal children. *Ann Neurol*, 1998, 43, 135-142.

[3] Morrish, E; King, MA; Smith, IE; Shneerson, JM. Factors associated with a delay in the diagnosis of narcolepsy. *Sleep Med*, 2004, 5, 37-41.

[4] Nevsimalova, S; Pretl, M; Vankova, J; Blazejova, K; Sonka, K. Narcolepsy in children and adolescents. In: P. Evrard, C. Richelme, & M. Tardieu (Eds.), *3rd EPNS Congress*. Bologna: Monduzzi, 1999, 73-77.

[5] Einen, MA; Aran, A; Mignot, E; Nishino, S. Pre-versus post-pubertal narcolepsy in children. *Sleep*, 2009, 32 (Suppl.), A249-A250.
[6] Dauvilliers, Y; Montplaisir, J; Molinari, N; Carlander, B; Ondze, B; Besset, A. et al. Age at onset of narcolepsy in two large populations of patients in France and Quebeck. *Neurology*, 2001, 57, 2029-2033.
[7] Ohayon, MM; Priest, RG; Zulley, J; Smirne, S; Paiva T. Prevalence of narcolepsy symptomatology and diagnosis in the European general population. *Neurology*, 2002, 58, 1826-1833.
[8] Silber, MH; Krahn, LE; Olson, EJ; Pankratz, VS. The epidemiology of narcolepsy in Olmsted County, Minnesota: A population-based study. *Sleep*, 2002, 25, 197-202.
[9] Challamel, MJ; Mazzola, ME; Nevšímalová, S; Cannard, C; Louis, J; Revol, S.; et al. *Sleep*, 1994, 17(Suppl 8), S17-S20.
[10] Dauvilliers, Y; Gosselin, A; Paquet, J; Touchon, J; Billiard, M; Montplaisir, J. Effect of age on MSLT results in patients with narcolepsy-cataplexy. *Neurology*, 2004, 62, 46-50.
[11] Nevsimalova, S; Buskova, J; Kemlink, D; Sonka, K; Skibova, J. Does age at the onset of narcolepsy influence the course and severity of the disease? *Sleep Med*, 2009, 10, 967-972.
[12] Mignot, E. Sleep, sleep disorder and hypocretin (orexin). *Sleep Med*, 2004, 5(Suppl 1), S2-S8.
[13] Kadotani, H; Faraco, J; Mignot, E. Genetic studies in the sleep disorder narcolepsy. *Genome Res*, September 5, 2007, 427-434, www.genome.org.
[14] Lecendreux, M; Maret, S; Bassetti, C; Mouren, MC; Taffin, M. Clinical efficacy of high-dose intravenous immunoglobulins near the onset of narcolepsy in a 10-year-old-boy. Letter to the Editor. *J Sleep Res*, 2003, 12, 1-2.
[15] Dauvilliers, Y; Carlander, B; River, F; Touchon, J; Tafti, M. Successful management of cataplexy with intravenous immunoglobulins at narcolepsy onset. *Ann Neurol*, 2004, 56, 905-908.
[16] Dauvillier, Y. Follow-up of four narcolepsy patients treated with intravenous immunoglobulins. Letter, American Neurological Association, 2006. Published by Wiley-Liss, Inc., through Wiley Subscription Service.
[17] Hecht, M; Lin, L; Kushida, CA; Umetsu, DT; Taheri, S; Einen, M; et al. Immunosuppression with prednisone in an 8-year-old boy with an acute onset of hypocretin deficiency/narcolepsy. *Sleep*, 2003, 26, 809-810.

[18] Hallmayer, J; Faraco, J; Ling, L; Hesselson, S; Winkelmann J; Kawashima, M;, Mayer, G; et al. Narcolepsy is strongly associated with the CR alpha locus. *Nature Gen*, 2009, 41, 708-711.

[19] Aran, A; Lin, L; Nevsimalova, S; Plazzi, G; Hong, SC; Weiner, K; Mignot, E. Elevated anti-streptococcal antibodies in patients with recent narcolepsy onse. *Sleep*, 2009, 32, 979-983.

[20] Peterson, PC; Husain, AM. Pediatric narcolepsy. *Brain Dev*, 2008, 30, 609-623.

[21] Challamel, MJ. Hypersomnia in children. In: Billiard M, (ed.) *Sleep-Physiology, Investigation and Medicine.* New York: Kluwer Academic/Plenum Publishers; 2003; 457-468.

[22] Nevsimalova, S. Narcolepsy in children and adolescents. In: C. Bassetti, M. Billiard, & E. Mignot (Eds.), *Narcolepsy and Hypersomnia* Informa Healthcare USA, 2007, 67-75.

[23] Nevsimalova, S. Narcolepsy in childhood. *Sleep Med Rev*, 2009, 13, 169-180.

[24] Serra, L; Montagna, P; Mignot, E; Lugaresi, E; Plazzi G. Cataplexy features in childhood narcolepsy. *Mov Dis*, 2008, 23, 858-865.

[25] Wise, MS. Childhood narcolepsy. *Neurology*, 1998, 50(Suppl 1), S37-S42.

[26] Nevsimalova, S; Roth, B; Zouhar, A; Zemanova, H. The occurrence of narcolepsy-cataplexy and periodic hypersomnia in early childhood. In: W. P. Koella, F. Obal, H. Schulz, & P. Wisser (Eds.), *Sleep '86.* Stuttgart – New York. Gustav Fisher Verlag, 1988:399-401.

[27] Guilleminault, C; Pelayo, R. Narcolepsy in children. A practical guide to its diagnosis, treatment and follow-up. *Paediatr Drug*, 2000, 2, 1-9.

[28] Droogleever-Fortuyn, H; Lappenschaar, M; Nienhuis, F; Furer, J; Hodiamont, P; Rijnders, C; Lammers, GJ; et al. Hypnagogic hallucinations and „psychotic" symptoms in narcolepsy: A comparison with control subjects and schizophrenic patiens. *Sleep*, 2009, 32 (Suppl.), A244-A245.

[29] International Clasification of Sleep Disorders. Diagnostic and Coding Manual. 2nd ed. Westchester, IL, USA: American Academy of Sleep Medicine; 2005.

[30] Stores, G; Montgomery, P; Wiggs, L. The psychosocial problems of children with narcolepsy and those with excessive daytime sleepiness of uncertain origin. *Pediatrics*, 2006, 118, 1116-1123.

[31] Nevsimalova, S; Prihodova, I; Kemlink, D; Ling, L; Mignot, E. REM behavior disorder (RBD) can be one of the first symptoms of childhood narcolepsy. *Sleep Med*, 2007, 8, 784-786.

[32] Cyrille, V; Arnulf, A. Narcolepsy with long sleep time: A specific entity? *Sleep*, 2009, 32 (Suppl.), A243-A244.

[33] Nevsimalova, S; Vankova, J; Pretl, M; Bruck, D. Narcolepsy in children and adolescents – Clinical and psychosocial aspects (in Czech). *Ces Slov Neurol Neurochir*, 2002, 65, 169-174.

[34] Dahl, RE; Holttum, J; Trubnick, L. A clinical picture of child and adolescent narcolepsy. *J Am Acad Child Adolesc Psychiatry*, 1994, 33, 834-841.

[35] Kotagal, S; Krahn, LE; Slocumb, N. A putative link between childhood narcolepsy and obesity. *Sleep Med*, 2004, 5, 147-150.

[36] Dahmen, N; Bierbrauer, J; Kasten, M. Increased prevalence of obesity in narcoleptic patients and relatives. *Eur Arch Psychiatry Clin Neurosci*, 2001, 251, 85-89.

[37] Kok, SW; Overeem, S; Visscher, TL; Lammers, GJ; Seidell, JC; Pijl, H. et al. Hypocretin deficiency in narcoleptic humans is associated with abnominal obesity. *Obes Res*, 2003, 11, 1147-1154.

[38] Lammers, GJ; Pijl, H; Iestra, J; Buunk, G; Meinders, AE. Spontaneous food choice in narcolepsy. *Sleep*, 1996, 19, 75-76.

[39] Schuld, A; Beitinger, PA; Dalal, M; Geller, F; Wetter, TC; Albert, ED; et al. Increased body mass index (BMI) in male narcoleptic patients, but not in HLA-DR2-positive healthy male volunteers. *Sleep Med*, 2002, 3, 335-339.

[40] Nishino, S; Ripley, B; Overeem, S; Nevsimalova, S; Lammers, GJ; Vankova, J; et al. Low cerebrospinal fluid hypocretin (orexin) and altered energy homeostasis in human narcolepsy. *Ann Neurol*, 2001, 50, 381-388.

[41] Beuckmann, CT; Yanagisawa, M. Orexins: from neuropeptides to energy homeostasis and sleep/wake regulation. *J Mol Med*, 2002, 80, 329-342.

[42] Crocker, A; Espana, RA; Papadopoulou, M; Saper, CB; Faraco, J; Sakurai, T; et al. Concomitant loss of dynorphin, NARP, and orexin in narcolepsy. *Neurology*, 2005, 65, 1184-1188.

[43] Arnulf, I; Lin, L; Zhang, J; Russel, J; Ripley, B; Einen M. et al. CSF versus serum leptin in narcolepsy: Is there an effect of hypocretin deficiency? *Sleep*, 2006, 29, 1017-1024.

[44] Chabas, D; Foulon, C; Gonzales; Nasr, M; Caen, OL; Willer, JC; et al. Eating disorder and metabolism in narcoleptic patients. *Sleep*, 2007, 30, 1267-1273.

[45] Plazzi, G; Parmeggiani, A; Mignot, E; Lin, L; Scano, MC; Posar, A; et al. Narcolepsy-cataplexy associated with precocious puberty. *Neurology*, 2006, 66, 1577-1579.

[46] Nishino, S; Kanbayashi, T. Symptomatic narcolepsy, cataplexy and hypersomnia, and their implication in the hypothalamic hypocretin/orexin system. *Sleep Med Rev*, 2005, 9, 269-310.

[47] Marcus, CL; Trescher, WH; Halbower, AC; Lutz, J. Secondary narcolepsy in children with brain tumors. *Sleep*, 2002, 25, 435-439.

[48] Vankova, J; Stepanova, I; Jech, R; Elleder, M; Ling, L; Mignot, E; et al. Sleep disturbance and hypocretin deficiency in Niemann-Pick disease type C. *Sleep*, 2003, 26, 427-430.

[49] Smit, LS; Lammers, GL; Catsman-Berrevoets, CE. Cataplexy leading to the diagnosis of Niemann-Pick disease. *Ped Neurol*, 2006, 35, 82-84.

[50] Bouvier, E; Arnulf, I; Claustrat, B; Kocher, L; Bastuji H; Lecendreux, M; et al. Do children with idiopathic narcolepsy have a long sleep time? *Sleep*, 2009, 32 (Suppl.), A97.

[51] Kotagal, S; Hartse, KM; Walch, JK. Characteristics of narcolepsy in preteenaged children. *Pediatrics*, 1990, 85, 205-209.

[52] Carskadon, MA; Dement, WC; Mitler, M.; Roth, T; Westbrook, P; Keenan, S. Guideliness for the Multiple Sleep Latency Test (MSLT): a standard measure of sleepiness. *Sleep*, 1986, 9, 519-524.

[53] Carskadon, MA; Harvey, K; Duke, P; Anders, TF; Litt, IF; Dement, WC. Pubertal change in daytime sleepiness. *Sleep*, 1980, 3, 453-460.

[54] Kotagal, S; Goulding, PM. The laboratory assessment of daytime sleepiness in childhood. *J Clin Neurophysiol*, 1996, 13, 208-218.

[55] Kubota, H; Kanbayashi, T; Tanabe, Y; Ito, M; Takanashi, J; Kohno, Y; et al. Decreased cerebrospinal fluid hypocretin-1 levels near the onset of narcolepsy in 2 prepubertal children. *Sleep*, 2003, 26, 555-557.

[56] Nevsimalova, S; Mignot, E; Šonka, K; Arrigoni, JL. Familial aspects of narcolepsy-cataplexy in the Czech Republic. *Sleep*, 1997, 20, 1021-1026.

[57] Nishino, S. Clinical and neurobiological aspects of narcolepsy. *Sleep Med*, 2007, 8, 373-399.

[58] Mignot, E; Lammers, GJ; Ripley, B; Okun, M; Nevsimalova, S; Overeem, S; et al. The role of cerebrospinal fluid hypocretin in the diagnosis of narcolepsy and other hypersomnias. *Arch Neurol*, 2002, 59, 1553-1562.

[59] Guilleminault, C; Fromherz, S. Narcolepsy. diagnosis and management. In: M. H. Kryger, T. Roth, & W. C. Dement (Eds.), *Principles and Practice of Sleep Medicine*, 4th Edition, Philadelphia: Elsevier Sounders, 2005, 780-790.

[60] Greenhil, LL; Pliszka, S; Dulcan, MK; Bernet, W; Arnold, V; Beitchman, J; et al. Practice parameter for the use of stimulant medication in the treatment of children, adolescents, and adults. *J Am Acad Child Adolesc Psychiatry*, 2002, 41 (Suppl.2), 26S-49S.

[61] Hood, BM; Harbord, MG. Paediatric narcolepsy: Complexities of diagnosis. *J Paediatr Child Health*, 2002, 38, 618-621.

[62] Ivanenko, A; Tauman, R; Gozal, D. Modafinil in the treatment of excessive daytime sleepiness in children. *Sleep Med*, 2003, 4, 579-582.

[63] Biederman, J; Swanson, JM; Wigal, SB; Boellner, SW; Earl, CQ; Lopez, FA. A comparison of once–daily and divided doses of modafinil in children with attention-deficit/hyperactivity disorder: a randomized, double-blind, and placebo-controlled study. *J Clin Psychiatry*, 2006, 67, 727-735.

[64] Murali, H; Kotagal, S. Off-label treatment of severe childhood narcolepsy-cataplexy with sodium oxybate. *Sleep*, 2006, 29, 1025-1020.

[65] Chen, W; Black, J; Call, P; Mignot, E. Late-onset narcolepsy presenting as rapidly progressing muscle weakness: response to plasmapheresis. *Ann Neurol*, 2005, 58, 489-490.

In: Nacrolepsy: Symptoms, Causes... ISBN: 978-1-60876-645-1
Editors: G. Santos et al. pp. 107-115

Chapter V

Narcolepsy: Changes in Memory and Attentional Abilities

Sergio Chieffi*[*], *Giovanni Messina, Vincenzo De Luca and Marcellino Monda
Department of Experimental Medicine, Section of Physiology,
Second University of Naples, Via Costantinopoli 16, 80138, Napoli, Italy.

Summary

Many patients with narcolepsy complain about cognitive problems, in addition to the characteristic symptoms of increased tiredness and sleepiness. Neuropsychological researches have mainly focused on memory and attentional abilities. In contrast to self-reports, standardized assessment of memory abilities yielded intact or mild deficit of short- and long- term memory. Conversely, attentional deficits are frequently reported mostly if attention has to be maintained over longer periods of time and if the tasks require a higher degree of cognitive control.

[*] Corresponding author: Dipartimento di Medicina Sperimentale, Sezione di Fisiologia, Via Costantinopoli 16, 80138 Napoli, Italy, E-mail: sergio.chieffi@unina2.it, Fax number: +39 +81 +5667500

Narcolepsy is a sleep disorder classically characterized by excessive daytime sleepiness. Other symptoms of the disease include cataplexy, sleep paralysis, hypnagogic hallucinations and disturbed nocturnal sleep. Many patients with narcolepsy, in addition to the characteristic symptoms of increased tiredness and sleepiness, complain about cognitive problems that may have negative consequences on activities of daily living and psychosocial interaction. Researches have been performed to examine if subjective impressions of cognitive dysfunction depend on the presence of true deficits, and in particular if memory and attentional deficits are present.

Early researches into the life effects of narcolepsy reported that subjective memory problems are of significant concern to this clinical population. In a study of 46 narcoleptic patients, Broughton and Ghanem [2] found that 21 (47.8%) of the patients stated that their memory had deteriorated since the onset of the illness, 20 (46.5%) reported no change in memory, and 2.3% reported that memory had improved. Further, the majority (71.4%) indicated that narcolepsy had mainly affected recall for recent events. In contrast, only 2 (4.7%) of matched controls subjects reported memory difficulties in the appropriate period of life. Subsequent studies led to similar findings [3,21,23]. Broughton et al. [3] carried out a cross-cultural study involving 180 patients from Asia, Europe, and North America. Authors [3] found that 88 (48.9%) of the patients reported their memory had worsened after onset of the disease. Again, memory for recent events was most often affected by narcolepsy. Indeed, of the 88 patients with subjective memory problems, impairment of recall 'mainly for recent events' (versus remote events, or both) was reported in 81.0%. Narcoleptics frequently noted a number of other symptoms which might relate to the memory problems, such as chronic excessive daytime sleepiness, difficulties in concentrating, and visual difficulties [3]. Rogers and Rosenberg [21] found that 16 (53.3%) of the patients reported memory deterioration since the onset of the symptoms as compared with 12 (40%) of the control subjects. Again, all the patients who reported subjective memory deterioration indicated that narcolepsy had mainly affected recall of recent events. Smith et al. [23] observed that 38% of the 700 interviewed narcoleptic reported moderate or severe memory problems, 39% had problems with forgetfulness, 40% with concentration and 26% with general learning processes. Hood and Bruck [12] re-evaluated more extensively the subjective experience of diminished memory function reported by narcoleptics, by exploring their metamemory profile. Authors [12] administered the Metamemory in Adulthood (MIA) scale, developed by Dixon and Hultsch [4], to narcoleptics, patients experiencing excessive daytime sleepiness, and controls. The results indicated that patients with narcolepsy had lower 'self efficacy' (i.e., subject's confidence) for memory performance than either of the comparison groups, despite there being no significant difference between groups in relation to 'knowledge based aspects' of memory functioning (i.e., subject's understanding of the way that memory processes work and how to utilize memory strategies to enhance memory function) [12]. This lowered self efficacy in narcolepsy was expressed through increased anxiety about memory function, decreased evaluations of memory capacity and increased perceptions of memory decline in relation to the comparison groups [12]. Hood and Bruck [12] suggested that the negative cognitive self evaluations of narcoleptics might arise as a consequence of global psychosocial adjustment difficulties. An elevations in global anxiety was also observed in narcoleptic patients by Stepanski et al. [24] and Kales et al. [14] using the MMPI.

In contrast to self-report findings, memory performance in narcoleptic patients did not differ from control in most standardized researches [1,21,23]. Aguirre et al. [1] were the first researchers to attempt an objective evaluation of the subjective experience of narcoleptics of diminished memory function. Authors [1] compared untreated narcoleptic patients, which expressed marked subjective memory difficulties, and matched controls, on a quite extensive battery of neuropsychological tests that assessed short-term memory, long-term memory, attention and concentration. No significant intergroup differences were found. Aguirre et al. [1] concluded that narcoleptics do not have a true organic memory deficit, but rather a subjective problem due to drowsiness which they are able to suppress during short testing sessions in a laboratory environment. The patients did, in fact, find the tests motivating and were able to remain alert throughout. In their normal everyday life, on the other hand, memory impairment might relate to inability to recall information which occurs during their frequent periods of decreased alertness in unchallenging situations [1]. The results obtained by Aguirre et al. [1] were confirmed by other Authors [21,23]. In Rogers and Rosenberg's study [21], narcoleptic patients, and matched control subjects, performed a battery of neuropsychological tests to assess both immediate and delayed recall, as well as verbal and visual memory. The results showed that in narcoleptic patients there was no objective evidence of memory impairment, so as there were no significant differences in scores between subjects (both patients and controls) who reported subjective memory deterioration and those who reported no change in memory function. Rogers and Rosenberg [21] proposed three hypotheses to account for this finding: (a) patients' complaints of memory loss are unfounded; (b) memory testing occurs in an artificial environment that prevents the expression of memory deficits. Tests usually take place in a laboratory or clinical setting where the patient is presented with information to learn without the distractions and conflicting demands that occur in the classroom, at work, or at home; (c) standardized tests of memory function fail to detect deterioration in certain aspects of memory function that patients consider important. In contrast, Henry et al. [10] found that unmedicated narcoleptics performed significantly worse than matched controls in memory tasks (word recall and incidental memory paradigm, i.e. estimation of frequency of occurrence). Henry et al. [10] proposed that a perceptual-encoding deficit, by diminishing the efficiency to which target stimuli are attended to and processed, may underlie the problems in memory. Mild verbal memory deficit and evidence of increased forgetting rate were found in narcoleptics on immediate and delayed free recall (after 30 min) of prose passage from the Wechsler Memory Scale [17]. Naumann et al. [17] proposed that verbal memory problems found in narcoleptic might be related to reduced encoding efficiency. For example, being cognitive resources utilized above all to monitor instable vigilance levels, this might compromise the semantic organization of story content and word lists [17].

To evaluate the potential impact of sleepiness on memory function, Hood and Bruck [11] manipulated arousal conditions for narcoleptic patients. Under 'sleepy' conditions narcoleptics demonstrated no performance deficits on routine memory tasks but significant decrements in performance on a complex task (Paced Auditory Serial Addition task) in which patients were required to retain information in short-term storage whereas performing parallel cognitive task. Hood and Bruck [11] suggested that complex processing situations perhaps approach more the everyday experience of memory function and it is this everyday perception of cognitive dysfunction that is reflected in the subjective experiences of narcoleptic patients. Successively, Hood and Bruck [13] examined whether also normal sleepers exposed to a deprivation protocol showed significant decrements in performance on the Paced Auditory Serial Addition task. To develop a subjective level of sleepiness that equated with that identified by patients with narcolepsy, normal sleepers required a 32-h deprivation protocol. However, this induced sleepiness in normal sleepers did not result in any significant decrement in complex performance, a finding that was in contrast to the performance decrement previously found in patients with narcolepsy and equivalent subjective sleepiness ratings. Hood and Bruck [13] concluded that there were significant differences in the impact of sleepiness on complex performance between non-pathological sleep-deprived subjects and patients with narcolepsy.

Not surprisingly, patients with narcolepsy are most often found to differ from healthy control in the areas of attention [7,16]. Attention is not a unitary function but is composed of several different, sometimes highly specific, components (including alertness, vigilance, selective and divided attention) which are responsible for the control of the flow of information in the cognitive system [15,18,19].

A decrease of vigilance, i.e. an inability to sustain full alertness during normal activity, is frequently reported as deficit associated to narcolepsy [5,6,8,9,22,25,26]. Valley and Broughton [25] carried out the first systematic study of vigilance performance in untreated narcoleptics and observed that narcoleptics performed significantly worse than matched controls on the more monotonous tests of auditory vigilance and the 4-choice serial RT, but not on tasks assessing rate of information processing and simple attention span. Similarly, on 1-hour Wilkinson Auditory Vigilance test narcoleptic patients performed significantly worse, by making response omissions and false positive responses, and spent significantly less time in wakefulness than controls [26]. Further, Valley and Broughton [26] found that moment-to-moment fluctuations in performance run in parallel with fluctuations in neurophysiological indicators of alertness. Findley et al. [5,6], to detect impaired vigilance, required to untreated narcoleptic patients to perform a task ("Steer Clear") that simulated, on computer, a long and monotonous highway drive. Narcoleptics performed more poorly on the test by hitting a higher percentage of obstacles than did control subjects and evidencing a robust linear vigilance decrement. Schulz and Wilde-Frenz [22], to assess fluctuations in vigilance, measured critical flicker fusion (CFF) at 15-min intervals for 10 hours in narcoleptic patients and matched healthy controls. The narcoleptics showed a marked instability of performance across the trials. They were unable to perform at a steady level through the day. Schulz and Wilde-Frenz [22] suggested that cognitive processes in narcoleptic patients are not impaired on a functional but only on a temporal level. The tiredness and episodes of sleepiness seem to be the main reason for cognitive impairments in narcolepsy [22]. This view was further supported by Schultz and Wilde-Frenz [22] who examined retrospectively narcoleptics' performance in neuropsychological tests. Authors [22] grouped the tests into those in which patients showed a performance deficit and those which did not. Schultz and Wilde-Frenz [22] found a rather consistent pattern: (a) narcoleptics patients displayed only very limited or no performance deficit if tests were short and challenging; (b) clear-cut differences between narcoleptics and healthy control were present when monotonous tasks with a low rate of information input and which lasted for an extended time period were performed, a situation which is typical for tests of vigilance [22].

Some Authors conducted a more systematic investigation of different aspects of attention in patients with narcolepsy [17,20]. Rieger et al. [20] examined changes in attentional abilities such as phasic alertness (i.e., the ability to increase the attentional level when a stimulus of high priority is likely to appear), focused attention (i.e., the ability to attend to relevant stimuli), divided attention (i.e., the ability to share attention between different source of information) and flexible attention (i.e., the ability to change the focus of attention). The results showed that narcoleptics had no deficit in phasic alertness and focused attention, but specific deficits occurred in divided attention, probably due to attentional capacity limitations, and flexible attention, probably due to attention control deficits. Further, narcoleptics had slower and more variable RTs so as observed in previous studies [8,22,25,26]. Rieger et al. [20] proposed that attentional deficit cannot solely be explained by impairments on the temporal level of attention, but other functions like attentional capacity and control are also impaired. Comparable findings were also reported by Naumann et al. [17]. Naumann et al. [17] performed a battery of neuropsychological tests to assess changes in attentional and executive functions. Attentional function tasks assessed the ability of narcoleptic patient across a range of attention system subcomponents, i.e. alertness, selective attention, divided attention and sustained attention/concentration. Executive function tasks assessed the ability to initiate responses, to suppress prepotent responses and the efficiency of strategy-guided access to verbal semantic memory. The results showed that narcoleptics and control did not differ significantly on alertness, selective attention and concentration tasks. On divided attention task narcoleptics did not differed from controls in terms of performance accuracy, but a slowing of information processing was present. Further, the performances of narcoleptics in executive function tasks were consistently impaired [17]. Naumann et al. [17] suggested that the slowing of attentional processes and the impairment of executive functions observed in those tasks which required higher demands could depend on a reduction or limitation of cognitive processing resources. A deficit of sustained attention was also observed by Rogers and Rosenberg [21]. Specifically, narcoleptic patients made significantly more perseveration error on Strub and Black's List of Letters than control [21].

Overall experimental evidence strongly suggests that altered sleep regulation mechanisms in narcolepsy, by inducing continuous fluctuations in vigilance and attention, may interfere with cognitive processes. Further, a deficit on cognitive performance occurs mostly when attention has to be maintained over longer periods of time and the task requires a higher degree of cognitive control. However, further investigations are necessary to understand in more detail the changes in cognitive abilities in narcoleptic patients.

References

[1] Aguirre, M., Broughton, R. & Stuss, D. (1985). Does memory impairment exist in narcolepsy-cataplexy? *J Clin Exp Neuropsychol*, *7*, 14-24.

[2] Broughton, R. & Ghanem Q. (1976). The impact on compound narcolepsy in the life of the patient. In C. Guilleminault, W. Dement, P. Passouant, & E. Weitzman (Eds.), Narcolepsy (Advances in sleep research, Vol. 3, 201–220). Holliswood, NY: Spectrum Publications.

[3] Broughton, R., Ghanem, Q., Hishikawa, Y., Sugita, Y., Nevsimalova, S. & Roth, B. (1981). Life effects of narcolepsy in 180 patients from North America, Asia and Europe compared to matched controls. *Can J Neurol Sci*, *8*, 299-304.

[4] Dixon, R. A. & Hultsch, D. F. (1983). Structure and development of metamemory in adulthood. *J Gerontol*, *38*, 682-8.

[5] Findley, L. J., Suratt, P. M. & Dinges, D. F. (1999). Time-on-task decrements in "steer clear" performance of patients with sleep apnea and narcolepsy. *Sleep*, *22*, 804-9.

[6] Findley, L., Unverzagt, M., Guchu, R., Fabrizio, M., Buckner, J. & Suratt, P. (1995). Vigilance and automobile accidents in patients with sleep apnea or narcolepsy. *Chest*, *108*, 619-24.

[7] Fulda, S. & Schulz, H. (2001). Cognitive dysfunction in sleep disorders. *Sleep Med Rev*, *5*, 423-445.

[8] Godbout, R. & Montplaisir, J. (1986). All-day performance variations in normal and narcoleptic subjects. *Sleep*, *9*, 200-4.

[9] Ha, K. S., Yoo, H. K., Lyoo, I. K. & Jeong, D. U. (2007). Computerized assessment of cognitive impairment in narcoleptic patients. *Acta Neurol Scand*, *116*, 312-6.

[10] Henry, G. K., Satz, P. & Heilbronner, R. L. (1993). Evidence of a perceptual-encoding deficit in narcolepsy? *Sleep*, *16*, 123-7.

[11] Hood, B. & Bruck, D. (1996). Sleepiness and performance in narcolepsy. *J Sleep Res*, *5*, 128-34.

[12] Hood, B. & Bruck, D. (1997). Metamemory in narcolepsy. *J Sleep Res*, *6*, 205-10.

[13] Hood, B. & Bruck, D. (2002). A comparison of sleep deprivation and narcolepsy in terms of complex cognitive performance and subjective sleepiness. *Sleep Med*, *3*, 259-66.

[14] Kales, A., Soldatos, C. R., Bixler, E. O., Caldwell, A., Cadieux, R. J., Verrechio, J. M. & Kales, J. D. (1982) Narcolepsy-cataplexy. II. Psychosocial consequences and associated psychopathology. *Arch Neurol*, *39*, 169-71.

[15] Lyon, G. R. & Krasnegor, N. A. (1996). *Attention, memory and executive function*. Baltimore: Paul H. Brookes.

[16] Naumann, A. & Daum, I. (2003). Narcolepsy: pathophysiology and neuropsychological changes. *Behav Neurol*, *14*, 89-98.

[17] Naumann, A., Bellebaum, C. & Daum, I. (2006). Cognitive deficits in narcolepsy. *J. Sleep Res*, *15*, 329-338.

[18] Posner, M. I. & Petersen, S. E. (1990). The attention system of the human brain. *Annu Rev Neurosci.*, *13*, 25-42.

[19] Posner, M. I. & Rafal, R. D. (1987). Cognitive theories of attention and the rehabilitation of attentional deficits. In: M. J. Meier, A. L. Benton, & L. Diller (Eds.), *Neuropsychological Rehabilitation* (182-201). Edinburgh: Churchill Livingston.

[20] Rieger, M., Mayer, G. & Gauggel, S. (2003). Attention deficits in patients with narcolepsy. *Sleep*, *26*, 36-43.

[21] Rogers, A. E. & Rosenberg, R. S. (1990). Tests of memory in narcoleptics. *Sleep*, *13*, 42-52.

[22] Schulz, H. & Wilde-Frenz, J. (1995). Symposium: Cognitive processes and sleep disturbances: The disturbance of cognitive processes in narcolepsy. *J Sleep Res*, *4*, 10-14.

[23] Smith, K. M., Merritt, S. M. & Cohen, F. L. (1992). Can We Predict Cognitive Impairments in Persons with Narcolepsy? *Loss Grief Care*, *5*, 103-133.

[24] Stepanski, E. J., Markey, J. J., Zorick, F. J. & Roth, T. (1990) Psychometric profiles of patient populations with excessive daytime sleepiness. *Henry Ford Hosp Med J*, *38*, 219-22.

[25] Valley, V. & Broughton, R. (1981). Daytime performance deficits and physiological vigilance in untreated patients with narcolepsy-cataplexy compared to controls. *Rev Electroencephalogr Neurophysiol Clin*, *11*, 133-9.

[26] Valley, V. & Broughton, R. (1983). The physiological (EEG) nature of drowsiness and its relation to performance deficits in narcoleptics. *Electroencephalogr Clin Neurophysiol*, *55*, 243-51.

In: Nacrolepsy: Symptoms, Causes...
Editors: G. Santos et al. pp. 117-122
ISBN: 978-1-60876-645-1

Chapter VI

Does Orexin A Control Wakefulness by an Influence on Body Temperature?

Marcellino Monda*, Giovanni Messina, Andrea Viggiano, Emanuela Viggiano and Vincenzo De Luca[*]
Department of Experimental Medicine, Section of Human Physiology and Clinical Dietetic Service, Second University of Naples, Via Costantinopoli 16, 80138 Naples, Italy.

Summary

Orexin A is produced almost exclusively in the dorsal and lateral hypothalamus but its projection is widespread within the brain and plays important roles. This system plays a crucial role in the regulation of sleep and wakefulness. On the other hand, orexin A exerts a strong influence on thermoregulation and eating behavior. This peptide could control sleep/wakefulness states throughout modifications of body temperature and eating behavior. The influences of orexin A in the pathophysiological mechanisms of narcolepsy are discussed.

[*] Corresponding author: Dipartimento di Medicina Sperimentale, Sezione di Fisiologia Umana e Servizio di Dietetica, Seconda Università di Napoli, Via Costantinopoli 16, 80138 Napoli, Italy, E-mail: marcellino.monda@unina2.it, Tel.: +39 +81 566 5823, Fax: +39 +81 5667500.

Sakurai et al. [20] described two novel neuropeptides that increased food intake when given to rodens. They were named "orexin-A" and "orexin-B," orexin coming from *orexis,* which refers to appetite. Contemporaneously De Lecea et al.[5] discovered two peptides: hypocretins. The name was coined from the word *hypo*thalamus, referring to the anatomic location of neurotransmitter, and se*cretin*, the gastric peptide with which hypocretin (Hcrt) was thought to share considerable homology. Using directional tag PCR subtraction, they discovered a hypothalamus-specific mRNA that was thought to encode the peptides Hcrt-1 and Hcrt-2. These peptides were restricted to neuronal bodies in the dorsal and lateral hypothalamus with fibers projecting to multiple targets in the hypothalamus, thalamus, and brainstem. Hypocretin and orexin are considered synonymous.

The presence of orexin receptors in many cerebral areas suggests that additional functions are played by orexin A [9, 11]. A role for the orexins in sleep regulation has also been demonstrated [1, 17]. In 1999, two American groups simultaneously published data linking the orexinergic system with narcolepsy. Mignot's group used positional cloning to identify an autosomal recessive mutation in one of the orexin receptor genes, orexin-receptor2, in narcoleptic canines [10]. Mutation analysis of 17 narcoleptic Doberman pinschers revealed the same insertion mutation in orexin-receptor2; the insertion was absent in all 36 comparison dogs tested. Ripley et al. [18] later showed that orexin ligand levels in the brain and cerebral spinal fluid of Doberman pinschers were within normal range, supporting the theory that in canines, narcolepsy develops as a result of a mutation in the receptor gene. The search for genetic alterations in human narcolepsy has demonstrated that orexin and orexin-receptor mutations are rare. This is not surprising as most human narcolepsy is not familial and is discordant in identical twins. The likely cause of narcolepsy in humans was found to be a degeneration of orexinergic system [24]. The neuronal loss was limited to orexin-neurons as melanin-concentrating hormone neurons, which are intermixed with orexin-cells, were unaffected. This raised the possibility of narcolepsy being a neurodegenerative disease such as Alzheimer's disease or Parkinson's disease. Despite strong evidence from animal and human studies that orexin plays a role in the development of narcoleptic symptoms, the exact pathophysiological link between orexin and narcolepsy in humans remains unclear. Changes in body temperature due to orexinergic activity could be a valid explanation of the link between orexin and narcolepsy. Indeed, orexin A affects strongly body temperature in a relevant manner so that the name "hyperthermin A" has been suggested instead of orexin A [12, 14, 15].

An intracerebroventricular administration of orexin A induces an increase in the firing rate of the sympathetic nerves to interscapular brown adipose tissue, accompanied with a strong rise in body temperatures [16]. Food intake is increased by orexin A, but this increase is reduced when food presentation is delayed, as demonstrated by the following experiment. Body temperature and food intake were monitored in 24h-fasting male Sprague-Dawley rats after an administration of orexin A. When the orexin injection and food presentation were contemporaneous, the amount of ingested food was significant higher than that measured after a delayed presentation of food. These findings demonstrate that the effects on food intake induced by orexin A depends on the time of food presentation [12]. This induces to revise the role of orexin A in the control of food intake. The name assigned to this peptides was due to the strong increase in food intake after an orexin A administration, assigning a fundamental role in the induction of food intake [20, 22, 25]. The results of the above mentioned experiment call for a re-discussion of this role, underlining the importance of orexin A in the control of body temperature, which in turn affects food intake. This suggests that the effects on thermoregulation are prevalent with respect to eating behavior. Then, orexin A can induce hyperphagia, but also hypophagia, contradicting the significance of this name that assign a primary hyperphagic effect to this peptide.

The influence of orexin A on body temperature are due to effects exerted on sympathetic activity. An intracerebroventricular injection of this hypothalamic neuropeptide is able to induce multiform reactions, as expression of generalized activation of sympathetic nervous system, including also an increase in heart rate [16] and blood pressure [23].

Although these effects are caused by activation of the sympathetic branch of the autonomic nervous system [2, 21], it is also possible that orexin A can influence the dorsal motor nucleus of the vagus nerve, which is a major parasympathetic center [4]. The ability of orexin A to stimulate sympathetic activity is fairly well established, however, some groups report depressor effects especially when orexin A is directly injected into other regions of the brain. De Oliveira et al.[6] report that orexin A in the nucleus tractus solitarus increases vagal activity to the heart and inhibits sympathetic activity. The same group reported similar findings with orexin A in the nucleus ambiguous [3]. These contradictory findings can be explained by the inherent limitation of in situ experiments with neurotransmitters. Site-specific delivery is not anatomically localized or functionally specific and does not represent true physiological conditions. In vivo experiments seem to indicate that orexin A has primarily a sympatho-stimulatory effect. Knockout mice deficient in orexins have a significantly lower mean arterial blood pressure (MAP) than normal mice. The difference in MAP in wild-type and mutant mice can be cancelled with α-adrenergic blockade and ganglionic blockade. These treatments lowered the MAP of wild-type mice significantly more than that of mutant mice resulting in MAPs that were statistically identical. Conversely, treatment with angiotensin-converting enzyme inhibition or vasopressin antagonism affected the MAP of both wild-type and mutant mice in a similar manner. This suggests that the cardiovascular status of the knockout mice is due to decreased sympathetic vasoconstrictor tone [7]. In human narcoleptics, subnormal heart rate, blood pressure, and forearm blood flow responses to muscle contraction are observed as well as subnormal heart rate response to the Valsalva maneuver [19].

Orexin A could control sleep/wakefulness states throughout modifications of body temperature due to changes in the sympathetic activity. The influence on the body temperature should be the primary action of orexin A, so that all other physiological changes should be secondary effects to maintain a correct body temperature. On the other words, orexin A modifies the hypothalamic thermal set-point, so that reactions due to an administration of orexin A serve to reach new thermo-neutral level. These reactions include vasoconstriction that serves to reduce heat dissipation, and wakefulness state that is aimed to increase motor activity [8] and food intake. These behavioral changes serve to elevate body temperature, in accord to an unifying view of physiological role exerted by orexin A.

The above reported demonstrations support the hypothesis that orexin A is a thermoregulatory peptide, which has a strong influence on sleep/awake cycle as a factor controlling body temperature. This view is useful in investigations of pathophysiological mechanisms of sleep disorders.

In addition, it is irrational to utilize a misleading name, as orexin A, for a thermoregulatory neuropeptide, so that we can insist to use a new nomenclature for this peptide. The name “hypertermine A” (already suggested some years ago) seen to be appropriated, because it is indicates the primary function. This name is more appropriate than hypocretin-1, which indicates the site of the synthesis, but not the physiological role.

References

[1] Borgland, SL; Taha, SA; Sarti, F; Fields, HL; Bonci, A. Orexin A in the VTA is critical for the induction of synaptic plasticity and behavioral sensitization to cocaine. *Neuron*, 2006, 49, 589-601.

[2] Chen, CT; Hwang, LL; Chang, JK. Pressor effects of orexins injected intracisternally and to rostral ventrolateral medulla of anesthetized rats. *Am J Physiol Regul Integr Comp Physiol*, 2000, 278, R692-697.

[3] Ciriello, J; de Oliveira, CV. Cardiac effects of hypocretin-1 in nucleus ambiguus. *Am J Physiol Regul Integr Comp Physiol*, 2003, 284, R1611-1620.

[4] Davis, SF; Williams, KW; Xu, W. Selective enhancement of synaptic inhibition by hypocretin (orexin) in rat vagal motor neurons: implications for autonomic regulation. *J Neurosci*, 2003, 23, 3844-3854.

[5] de Lecea, L; Kilduff, TS; Peyron, C. The hypocretins: hypothalamus-specific peptides with neuroexcitatory activity. *Proc Natl Acad Sci*, USA, 1998, 95, 322-327.

[6] de Oliveira, CV; Rosas-Arellano, MP; Solano-Flores, LP. Cardiovascular effects of hypocretin-1 in nucleus of the solitary tract. *Am J Physiol Heart Circ Physiol*, 2003, 284, H1369-1377.

[7] Kayaba, Y; Nakamura, A; Kasuya, Y. Attenuated defense response and low basal blood pressure in orexin knockout mice. *Am J Physiol Regul Integr Comp Physiol*, 2003, 285, R581-593.

[8] Kotz, CM. Integration of feeding and spontaneous physical activity: role for orexin. *Physiol Behav*, 2006, 88, 294-301.

[9] Kukkonen, JP; Holmqvist, T; Ammoun, S; Akerman, KE. Functions of the orexinergic/hypocretinergic system. *Am J Physiol*, 2002, 283, C1567-1591.

[10] Lin, L; Faraco, J; Li, R. The sleep disorder canine narcolepsy is caused by a mutation in the hypocretin (orexin) receptor 2 gene. *Cell*, 1999, 98, 365-376.

[11] Marcus, JN; Aschkenasi, CJ; Lee, CE; Chemelli, RM; Saper, CB; Yanagisawa, M. Differential expression of orexin receptors 1 and 2 in the rat brain. *J Comp Neurol*, 2001, 435, 6-25.

[12] Monda, M; Viggiano, A; De Luca, V. A paradoxical effect of orexin A: the hypophagia induced by hyperthermia. *Brain Res*, 2003, 961, 220-228.

[13] Monda, M; Viggiano, A; Mondola, P; De Luca, V. Inhibition of prostaglandin synthesis reduces hyperthermic reactions induced by hypocretin-1/orexin A. *Brain Res*, 2001, 909, 68-74.

[14] Monda, M; Viggiano, An; Viggiano, Al; Fuccio, F; De Luca V. Cortical spreading depression blocks the hyperthermic reaction induced by orexin A. *Neuroscience*, 2004, 123, 567-574.

[15] Monda, M; Viggiano, A; Viggiano, A; Viggiano, E; De Luca, V. Risperidone potentiates the sympathetic and hyperthermic reactions induced by orexin A in the rat. *Physiol Res*, 2006, 55, 73-78.

[16] Monda, M; Viggiano, An; Viggiano, Al; Viggiano, E; Lanza, A; De Luca, V. Hyperthermic reactions induced by orexin A: role of the ventromedial hypothalamus. *Eur J Neurosci*, 2005, 22, 1169-1175.

[17] Ohno, K; Sakurai, T. Orexin neuronal circuitry: role in the regulation of sleep and wakefulness. *Front Neuroendocrinol*, 2008, 29, 70-87.

[18] Ripley, B; Fujiki, N; Okura, M. Hypocretin levels in sporadic and familial cases of canine narcolepsy. *Neurobiol Dis*, *2001*, 8, 525-534.

[19] Sachs, C; Kaijser, L. Autonomic regulation of cardiopulmonary functions in sleep apnea syndrome and narcolepsy. *Sleep*, 1982, 5, 227-238.

[20] Sakurai, T; Amemiya, A; Ishii, M. Orexins and orexin receptors: a family of hypothalamic neuropeptides and G protein-coupled receptors that regulate feeding behavior. *Cell*, 1998, 92, 573-585.

[21] Samson, WK; Gosnell, B; Chang, JK. Cardiovascular regulatory actions of the hypocretins in brain. *Brain Res*, 1999, 831, 248-253.

[22] Shiraishi, T; Oomura, Y; Sasaki, K; Wayner, MJ. Effects of leptin and orexin-A on food intake and feeding related hypothalamic neurons. *Physiol Behav*, 2000, 71, 251-261.

[23] Shirasaka, T; Nakazato, M; Matsukura, S; Takasaki, M; Kannan, H. Sympathetic and cardiovascular actions of orexins in conscious rats. *Am J Physiol*, 1999, 277, R1780-R1785.

[24] Thannickal, TC; Moore, RY; Nienhuis, R. Reduced number of hypocretin neurons in human narcolepsy. *Neuron*, 2000, 27, 469-474.

[25] Wolf, G. Orexins: a newly discovered family of hypothalamic regulators of food intake. *Nutr Rev*, 1998, 56, 172-173.

In: Nacrolepsy: Symptoms, Causes...
Editors: G. Santos et al. pp. 123-128
ISBN: 978-1-60876-645-1

Chapter VII

Periodic Leg Movements in Narcolepsy

Ahmed Bahammam *

Sleep Disorders Center, College of Medicine, King Saud University, Riyadh, Saudi Arabia.

Abstract

The causes of sleep disruption in patients with narcolepsy are not clearly identified. Possible causes include daytime sleep through planned or unplanned naps, impairment of the delta-wave generating mechanisms, and comorbid sleep disorders such as sleep disordered breathing and periodic leg movements (PLMs). PLMs have been proposed as one of the causes of increased arousal in narcolepsy. Two recent controlled studies have demonstrated increased prevalence of PLMs in narcoleptics compared to controls with an impact on sleep latency on multiple sleep latency test. At the present, the contribution of PLMs to the perceived sleep quality and daytime sleepiness in narcolepsy patients is not clear. The observation that PLMs arousals were significantly higher in the PLMs group suggests that reducing the frequency of PLMs may improve sleep architecture. The pathophysiology of narcolepsy may involve an abnormal cholinergic-

* Corresponding Author: Sleep Disorders Center, College of Medicine, King Saud University, P. O. Box 225503, Riyadh 11324, Saudi Arabia, E-mail: ashammam2@gmail.com; ashammam2@yahoo.com, Telephone: 966-1-467-9179, Fax: 966-1-467-9495

dopaminergic interaction. Pharmacological agents that decrease dopaminergic release, such as gamma-hydroxybutyrate and neuroleptic-D2 receptor antagonists, have been shown to worsen PLMs. Additionally, dysfunction in the hypocretin/dopaminergic system is likely to be one of the mechanisms involved in the pathophysiology of narcolepsy, with alterations in arousal systems but also in sleep-related motor activation with a large amount of PLMS.

Introduction

Although narcoleptics usually have normal duration of nocturnal sleep, they have also been found to have nocturnal sleep disruptions, during which they have an increased number of awakenings, increased wake-time after sleep onset, increased time in stage 1 sleep and rapid eye movement (REM) sleep fragmentation.[1, 2] The causes of sleep disruption in patients with narcolepsy are not clearly identified. Possible causes include daytime sleep through planned or unplanned naps, impairment of the delta-wave generating mechanisms,[3] and comorbid sleep disorders such as sleep disordered breathing and periodic leg movements (PLMs). PLMs have been proposed as one of the causes of increased arousal in narcolepsy. PLMs have been shown to be more prevalent in narcoleptics than in the general population or in patients with idiopathic hypersomnia.[4-7] PLMs are rhythmical extensions of the great toe and partial flexion of the ankle, knee and hip that last 0.5-5 seconds and occur at a frequency of once every 5-90 seconds.[8] However, other muscles can be involved. PLMs during sleep occur in 6-13% of the general population, either as an isolated phenomenon or with other sleep disorders.[9-11] PLMs were first documented polygraphically in the restless legs syndrome (RLS).[12] While some investigators consider PLMs as simple polysomnographic occurrences that do not affect sleep architecture in most subjects,[13] others regard the assessment of PLMs as an essential component of an overnight sleep study.[14]

Prevalence of PLMs in Narcolepsy Patients

Recently, in a controlled study (age, male-to-female ratio and body mass index matched normal controls) in 47 newly diagnosed narcolepsy patients, we reported a prevalence of PLMs index $\geq$ 5/hr in 66% of narcolepsy patients and have shown that narcolepsy patients with PLMs have a higher arousal index and increased PLM arousals (during REM and NREM sleep) compared with narcolepsy patients without PLMs.[5] Additionally, we observed a significant correlation between PLM index and arousal index, stage shifts, and stage 1 and a negative correlation with average sleep latency on multiple sleep latency test (MSLT) but no differences in the EEG absolute power during NREM sleep of daytime naps. Dauvilliers et al reported similar findings in a recent controlled study.[7] They reported a prevalence of PLMs ≥5/hr of sleep in 67% of narcoleptics compared to 37% of controls and an index ≥10 (53% versus 21%).[7] Despite the fact that PLMs indices were higher in narcoleptics in both NREM and REM sleep compared to controls; the difference was more obvious in REM sleep.[7] Two-thirds of patients with narcolepsy had PLMs index in REM sleep > 5/hr compared with only one third of the controls.[7]

It is important for the reader to realize that studies addressing the prevalence and effects of PLMS on sleep architecture in narcoleptics are limited and have given conflicting results. Earlier studies, which defined PLMs as ≥100 leg movements per night, showed relatively lower prevalence.[15] More recent studies, which used a PLMS index of ≥5/hr, showed higher prevalence rates.[5, 7, 16] Additionally, conflicting results have been reported on the effects of PLMs on sleep architecture in narcolepsy patients, with some researchers concluding that PLMs disturb sleep [2] and others concluding that they do not.[1] Using a large cohort of 530 patients, Harsh et al found that narcolepsy patients with PLM index ≥5/hr have poorer sleep, with greater arousal, awakening and awake >2 min indices, enhanced stage 1 and reduced sleep efficiency. [2] However, the group with PLMs index ≥5/hr were significantly older than the group with PLMS index <5/hr, which may partially account for the elevated PLMS and the disturbed sleep architecture.[2] Another study found that narcolepsy patients with PLMS were significantly older than those without PLMs.[1] When the groups were matched for age, however, the only difference was an increase in shifts from stage 2 to stage 1 or waking in the PLMS group.[1] Hence it is important to control for the age when studying the prevalence and effects of PLMs in narcolepsy patients. In BaHammam's and Dauvilliers' et al studies, age-matched narcoleptics with and without PLMs were compared.[5, 7] Both studies demonstrated clearly that age-matched narcoleptics with PLMs had higher arousals than those without PLMs.[5, 7]

Impact of PLMs in Narcolepsy Patients

At the present, the contribution of PLMs to the perceived sleep quality and daytime sleepiness in narcolepsy patients is no clear. The observation that PLMs arousals were significantly higher in the PLMs group suggests that reducing the frequency of PLMs may improve sleep architecture.

The association between narcolepsy and PLMs and the fact the PLMs in narcoleptics are associated with shorter sleep latency in MSLT,[5, 7] raise the question of whether treating PLMs would result in improved sleep architecture in narcoleptics. Following treatment of narcoleptics with bromocriptine or L-dopa, the frequency of PLMs was reduced, without significant changes in sleep organization.[17, 18] When narcoleptics were treated with L-dopa, however, there was an improvement in daytime vigilance.[19] These conflicting results suggest that further studies are needed to determine the effects of new treatment modalities for PLMs on sleep architecture in narcoleptics.

Pathophysiology of PLMs in Narcolepsy

The pathophysiology of narcolepsy may involve an abnormal cholinergic-dopaminergic interaction.[20] Pharmacological agents that decrease dopaminergic release, such as gamma-hydroxybutyrate and neuroleptic-D2 receptor antagonists, have been shown to worsen PLMs.[21] Additionally, it is known that narcolepsy is characterized by a state of hypocretin deficiency.[22] Dopaminergic abnormalities are critical downstream mediators of the hypocretin deficiency.[23] Dysfunction in the hypocretin/dopaminergic system is likely to be one of the mechanisms involved in the pathophysiology of narcolepsy, with alterations in arousal systems but also in sleep-related motor activation with a large amount of PLMs.[7]

Conclusion

PLMs are prevalent in narcolepsy patients during sleep in both REM and NREM sleep. Patients with narcolepsy also show a specific increase of PLMs during REM sleep, which supports data indicating REM sleep disruption in this condition. Narcolepsy patients with PLMs have a higher arousal index and increased PLM arousals compared with narcolepsy patients without PLMs. Additionally, PLMs may increase daytime sleepiness in narcolepsy patients. Obviously, large studies, using large numbers of individuals, are needed to assess the impact of PLMs on sleep architecture in narcoleptics, the effects of different PLMs treatments on sleep architecture and daytime vigilance in narcoleptics and the common pathophysiological mechanisms underlying both disorders.

References

[1] Montplaisir, J; Godbout, R. Nocturnal sleep of narcoleptic patients: revisited. *Sleep*, 1986, 9(1 Pt 2), 159-61.

[2] Harsh, J; Peszka, J; Hartwig, G; Mitler, M. Night-time sleep and daytime sleepiness in narcolepsy. *J Sleep Res*, 2000, 9(3), 309-16.

[3] Guilleminault, C; Heinzer, R; Mignot, E; Black, J. Investigations into the neurologic basis of narcolepsy. *Neurology*, 1998, 50(2 Suppl 1), S8-15.

[4] Baker, TL; Guilleminault, C; Nino-Murcia, G; Dement, WC. Comparative polysomnographic study of narcolepsy and idiopathic central nervous system hypersomnia. *Sleep*, 1986, 9(1 Pt 2), 232-42.

[5] Bahammam, A. Periodic leg movements in narcolepsy patients: impact on sleep architecture. *Acta Neurol Scand*, 2007, 115(5), 351-5.

[6] BaHammam, A. Prevalence and impact of periodic leg movements in narcolepsy patients. *J Sleep Res*, 2009, 18(1), 142.

[7] Dauvilliers, Y; Pennestri, MH; Petit, D; Dang-Vu, T; Lavigne, G; Montplaisir, J. Periodic leg movements during sleep and wakefulness in narcolepsy. *J Sleep Res*, 2007, 16(3), 333-9.

[8] American Academy of Sleep Medicine. *International classification of sleep disorders*, 2nd edition: Diagnostic and coding manual. Westchester. IL: American Academy of Sleep Medicine, 2005.

[9] Coleman, RM; Roffwarg, HP; Kennedy, SJ; et al. Sleep-wake disorders based on a polysomnographic diagnosis. A national cooperative study. *JAMA*, 1982, 247(7), 997-1003.

[10] Bixler, EO; Kales, A; Vela-Bueno, A; Jacoby, JA; Scarone, S; Soldatos, CR. Nocturnal myoclonus and nocturnal myoclonic activity in the normal population. *Res Commun Chem Pathol Pharmacol*, 1982, 36(1), 129-40.

[11] Ohayon, MM; Roth, T. Prevalence of restless legs syndrome and periodic limb movement disorder in the general population. *J Psychosom Res*, 2002, 53(1), 547-54.
[12] Lugaresi, E; Coccagna, G; Tassinari, CA; Ambrosetto, C. [Polygraphic data on motor phenomena in the restless legs syndrome]. *Riv Neurol*, 1965, 35(6), 550-61.
[13] Mahowald, MW. Con: assessment of periodic leg movements is not an essential component of an overnight sleep study. *Am J Respir Crit Care Med*, 2001, 164(8 Pt 1), 1340-1, discussion 1-2.
[14] Walters, AS. Pro: assessment of periodic leg movements is an essential component of an overnight sleep study. *Am J Respir Crit Care Med*, 2001, 164(8 Pt 1), 1339-40.
[15] Wittig, R; Zorick, F; Piccione, P; Sicklesteel, J; Roth, T. Narcolepsy and disturbed nocturnal sleep. *Clin Electroencephalogr*, 1983, 14(3), 130-4.
[16] Montplaisir, J; Michaud, M; Denesle, R; Gosselin, A. Periodic leg movements are not more prevalent in insomnia or hypersomnia but are specifically associated with sleep disorders involving a dopaminergic impairment. *Sleep Med*, 2000, 1(2), 163-7.
[17] Boivin, DB; Lorrain, D; Montplaisir, J. Effects of bromocriptine on periodic limb movements in human narcolepsy. *Neurology*, 1993, 43(10), 2134-6.
[18] Boivin, DB; Montplaisir, J; Poirier, G. The effects of L-dopa on periodic leg movements and sleep organization in narcolepsy. *Clin Neuropharmacol*, 1989, 12(4), 339-45.
[19] Boivin, DB; Montplaisir, J. The effects of L-dopa on excessive daytime sleepiness in narcolepsy. *Neurology*, 1991, 41(8), 1267-9.
[20] Boutrel, B; Koob, GF. What keeps us awake: the neuropharmacology of stimulants and wakefulness-promoting medications. *Sleep*, 2004, 27(6), 1181-94.
[21] Montplaisir, J; Lorrain, D; Godbout, R. Restless legs syndrome and periodic leg movements in sleep: the primary role of dopaminergic mechanism. *Eur Neurol*, 1991, 31(1), 41-3.
[22] Mignot, E; Lammers, GJ; Ripley, B; et al. The role of cerebrospinal fluid hypocretin measurement in the diagnosis of narcolepsy and other hypersomnias. *Arch Neurol*, 2002, 59(10), 1553-62.
[23] Dauvilliers, Y; Billiard, M; Montplaisir, J. Clinical aspects and pathophysiology of narcolepsy. *Clin Neurophysiol*, 2003, 114(11), 2000-17.

In: Nacrolepsy: Symptoms, Causes...
Editors: G. Santos et al. pp. 129-132
ISBN: 978-1-60876-645-1

Chapter VIII

Body Weight Control and Narcolepsy

Marcellino Monda**, Messina Giovanni, Sergio Chieffi and Bruno De Luca
Department of Experimental Medicine, Section of Human Physiology and Clinical Dietetic Service, Second University of Naples, Via Costantinopoli 16, 80138 Naples, Italy.

Summary

This expert commentary reports the role exerted by obesity in the pathophysiological mechanisms of narcolepsy. Generally, the narcolepsy is described almost exclusively a neurological disease, while the role of nutritional and metabolic factors is almost neglected. The influences of body weight control and obesity are not sufficiently underlined. A search on "PubMed" (April 2009) with the words "narcolepsy and obesity" reports only 137 articles, while the search of the words "narcolepsy and body weight" produces 93 papers. This commentary underlines the importance of body weight as factor influencing the narcolepsy, indicating also the possible therapeutic strategies by modifications of eating behavior.

* Corresponding author: Dipartimento di Medicina Sperimentale, Sezione di Fisiologia Umana e Servizio di Dietetica, Seconda Università di Napoli, Via Costantinopoli 16, 80138 Napoli, Italy, E-mail: marcellino.monda@unina2.it, Tel.: +39 +81 566 5823, Fax: +39 +81 5667500.

The incidence of obesity is constantly growing in the rich populations and the World Health Organization considers the obesity as a “pandemia”. Body weight of 35-40% of American [2] and Southern European [1, 5] subjects is superior to normal value. Investigations into the mechanisms that control food intake and energy expenditure give growing relevance to the possibilities of new strategies to reduce the incidences of overweight and obesity, which are frequently associated with metabolic, cardiovascular and neurological diseases.

The narcolepsy is described almost exclusively a neurological disease [6], while the role of nutritional and metabolic factors is almost neglected. The influences exerted by overweight and obesity are undervalued. A search on “PubMed” (April 2009) with the words “narcolepsy and obesity” reports only 137 articles, while the search of the words “narcolepsy and body weight” produces 93 papers. Despite the scarcity of papers regarding narcolepsy and obesity, body weight is an important factor in the determination of sleep disorders. For example, body weight gain affects a sleep respiratory disorders, as nocturnal apnea, and narcolepsy, which is frequently associated to this respiratory disorder. Collapsible pharyngeal airway size is determined by interaction between structural properties of the pharyngeal airway and neural regulation of the pharyngeal dilating muscles. Obesity has two distinct mechanical influences on the pharyngeal airway collapsibility. First, obesity increases soft tissue surrounding the pharyngeal airway within limited maxillomandible enclosure occupying and narrowing its space (pharyngeal anatomical imbalance). Second, obesity, particularly central obesity, increases visceral fat volume decreasing lung volume. Pharyngeal wall collapsibility is increased by the lung volume reduction, possibly through decreased longitudinal tracheal traction (lung volume hypothesis). Neural compensation for functioning structural abnormalities operating during wakefulness is lost during sleep, leading to pharyngeal obstruction. Instability of the negative feedback of the respiratory system may accelerate cycling of pharyngeal closure and opening. Improvement of the pharyngeal anatomical imbalance and maintenance of lung volume are the keys for managements of obese patients with obstructive sleep apnea [3].

On the other hand, nocturnal apnea is not due only mechanical factors as increased abdominal mass and reduced lung volume, but also to metabolic factors. Then, sleep apnea is not "local abnormality" of the respiratory track, but it is a "systemic illness". Indeed, the beneficial effect of anti-inflammatory drugs and weight loss on excessive daytime sleepiness and apnea in obese subjects supports the hypothesis that cytokines and insulin resistance are mediators of some sleep disorders in humans [7].

The alterations in normal sleep/awake cycle due to visceral obesity induce modification of wakefulness periods and reduction of energy expenditure due to a decrease in motor activity. The reduction of physical activity is a determinant factor in the induction of body weight gain due to a fall in muscle energy expenditure. Decreased times spent in motor activity is noted in animal models utilized for investigations on narcolepsy. Indeed, narcolepsy of orexin knock-out rats is associated to body weight gain (despite reduced food intake) and reduced motor activity [4]. This experimental model underlines the link between body weight alterations and narcolepsy.

The reduction of body weight should be an important therapeutic tool to decrease abdominal mass and increase the lung capacity, so that the episodes of apnea could be reduced. Since there is a strict association between apnea and narcolepsy, the dietetic strategies to report body weight to normal values is essential in the therapy of these disorders.

In conclusion, more attention should be addressed to investigations regarding the influence of body weight on narcolepsy and other sleep disorders, so that dietetic schemes and appropriate exercise programs could be suggested to narcoleptic obese patients. Furthermore, the prevention of obesity could be considered as an important strategy to prevent sleep disorders or, at least, to slacken the progression of these diseases.

References

[1] Berghöfer, A; Pischon, T; Reinhold, T; Apovian, CM; Sharma, AM; Willich SN. Obesity prevalence from a European perspective: a systematic review. *BMC Public Health*, 2008, 8, 200-209.

[2] Brown, WV; Fujioka, K; Wilson, PW; Woodworth, KA. Obesity: why be concerned? *Am J Med*, 2009, 122, S4-11.

[3] Isono, S. Obstructive sleep apnea of obese adults: pathophysiology and perioperative airway management. *Anesthesiology*, 2009, 110, 908-921.

[4] Kaur, S; Thankachan, S; Begum, S; Blanco-Centurion, C; Sakurai, T; Yanagisawa, M; Shiromani, PJ. Entrainment of temperature and activity rhythms to restricted feeding in orexin knock out mice. *Brain Res*, 2008, 1205, 47-54.

[5] Leite, ML; Nicolosi, A. Dietary patterns and metabolic syndrome factors in a non-diabetic Italian population. *Public Health Nutr*, 2009, 15, 1-10.

[6] Panossian, LA; Avidan, AY. Review of sleep disorders. *Med Clin North Am*, 2009, 93, 407-425.

[7] Vgontzas, AN. Does obesity play a major role in the pathogenesis of sleep apnea and its associated manifestations via inflammation, visceral adiposity, and insulin resistance? *Arch Physiol Biochem*, 2008, 114, 211-223.

Index

A

C

E

F

G

H

I

J

K

L

M

N

O

P

T

U